I0789252

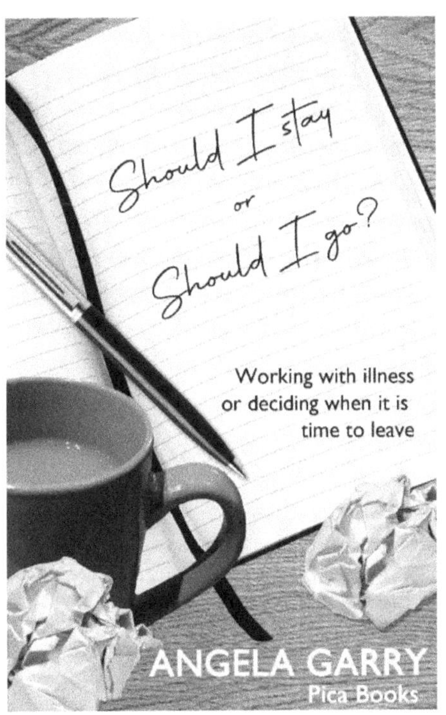

Should I stay
or
Should I go?
Working with illness
or deciding when it is
time to leave
ANGELA GARRY
Pica Books

Should I stay or should I go?

**Working with illness or deciding when it is
time to leave**

First published by Pica Books. Pica Books is wholly owned by
Angela Garry. www.picabooks.co.uk

First published 2021.

British Library Cataloguing-in-Publication Data:
A catalogue entry for this book is available from the British
Library.

ISBN: 978-1973795667

Printed and bound by Kindle Direct Publishing (KDP)

Dedication

To anyone in this most awkward of positions –

Good luck.

I've been there myself.

And I can report that it is possible to
come out safely the other side.

Acknowledgements

I'd like to offer my profound thanks to Professor Mary John, Colin Hetherington, Brian Byrne and Dave Harris – and in memoriam to Dr Stephen Bird, Brian Richardson and Dr E. Sarah Burnett (may you rest in peace).

You were, each and every one of you, the best bosses I could have wished to work for. Each of you, in your own inimitable ways, encouraged me to move onwards and upwards in my career, pushing, inspiring and challenging me - and I am forever grateful. You instilled faith and confidence in me that I could do whatever I set out to do. This allowed me to be brave enough to make my own decision on whether I should stay or go from my full-time job in education in 2014.

My thanks go to all the individuals who have shared their work-related illness / disability stories directly with me – and have consented for them included in this book.

Thanks also to my dear friends Marie Crowley and Jill Hughes for emotional and motivational support during the writing process for this book – and to Marie for putting me in touch with Aly Campbell and Ossian Hawkes at Ingeus, who kindly shared a number of case studies from the EA in IAPT programme.

Thank you all. xx

*Some names within the case studies have been changed to preserve privacy.

Contents

Introduction

It is commonly believed that as adults we should be working throughout our adult lives, but that doesn't mean we always can.

There are some who—for whatever health reason—absolutely cannot work. There are others who—despite their health issues—continue to work because they have no other choice.

And then there are those who continue to work, whilst sick and invisible, because they want to or because they still can. In some cases, this may unfortunately be slowly making them sicker. They may feel trapped, but feel that there are no other options open to them.

Whether we become chronically ill or injured, suffer mental health difficulties or become disabled, this means adjusting our life to accommodate our new levels of health and fitness, mentally and physically.

If you are reading this book it is because you are wondering about either continuing to work or quitting your job.

This is not a decision which can be made lightly, and there can be many social, financial, mental and physical implications and potential risks involved.

This book is designed for anyone who has acquired an illness, injury, mental health problem or disability that makes it difficult to stay in their current job without making some big changes.

These could include changes to your role, what you do, the hours you work, how you work them, where you work them, whether you work, what you earn, whether you earn at all, whether you stay or whether you go.

Continuing to work has social and financial benefits that may contribute towards your recovery. There are several ways you could maintain the different aspects of work:

- Change jobs to something you feel you are more able to do
- Reduce your hours or ask for the flexibility to change your hours when you need to
- Work from home
- Volunteer.

However, giving up work may be the best option for your health, especially if you are likely to be too ill to work long term.

Deciding to leave work is a big decision that effects not only your current finances but also those in the future. Therefore, it is advisable to take financial and legal advice alongside the advice of your doctor before you make the decision and give yourself enough time to do so after diagnosis.

Depending on where you live you may be legally protected – within the UK for example, the Equality Act and the Disability Discrimination Act protect against discrimination because of a medical diagnosis. This means a person cannot be advised by their employer to leave work for health reasons, especially within the first 12 months of them being ill.

You may want to continue working as you feel you are indispensable in your role and that your boss and the organisation – or your colleagues and those you manage – would never survive without you. If you are on sick leave at the moment though, they are doing just that.

Can you survive without your boss / the company?

Let's find out....

Each section in this book contains a number of questions to help you think about your illness, injury or disability as a whole. Some sections also contain some additional thinking points.

Having been through the "should I stay or go" process myself, I hope that this book – which includes all the questions I asked myself, plus some more besides – will help you towards your decision.

The questions encourage you to look closely at how your illness, injury, mental health or disability affects your job and your home life, your financial status, and your mental health and wellbeing, in order to help you to make your ultimate decision.

Along the way, you can expect to have to put on your mathematical head at times to add up the actual costs of staying or going – and your hypothetical head in terms of "what if I did this... or that....?" – plus you need to listen to what your heart, and your body, is telling you.

Whatever you choose to do, it's your journey – you need to make sure you are well equipped for it. I'd like to think that you wouldn't set out on a 5,000 mile road trip without having checked the oil, the tyre pressure, the water in the washers, the fuel, and at least looked at a map to plan your trip. It's only right that you should do the same when deciding the direction in which you want your future to go.

Use the questions in this book to examine the pros and the cons, the shoulds and the shouldn'ts, the oughts and the ought nots, the maybes, the whys, the wherefores, and most importantly the why nots, to help you decide.

At the end of the book I have included a range of personal experiences from a number of people (including me) about our own illnesses or disabilities and how these affected our ability to work.

Please remember: I'm not telling you what to decide. I have absolutely NO IDEA what it best for you.

This book is aimed to give you the tools to find out for yourself, and so that you can make an informed decision about what to do with your future.

I wish you all the very best of in whatever you choose to do – whether you choose to stay or go.

Angela Garry

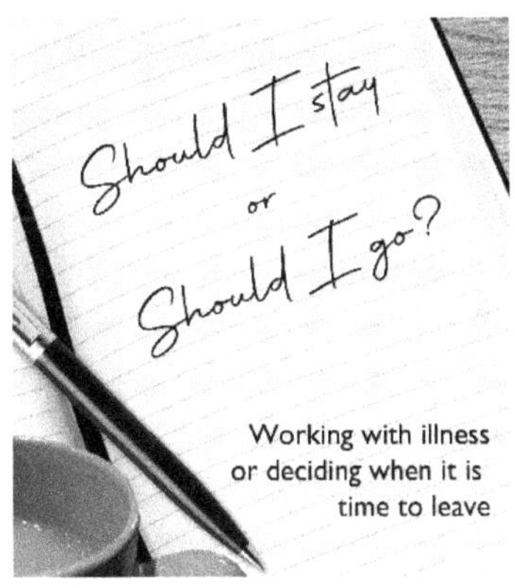

Questions about your illness / injury / disability

What is your illness / injury / disability, and how does it affect you?

- What is it?
- Do you have a name for your condition?
- How long have you had it?
- Have you been officially diagnosed by a doctor?
- What medications / treatments are you on?

What is your level of knowledge about your illness / injury / disability?

- What do you know about it?
- How much have you been told by medical professionals about your illness / injury / disability?
- What questions do you have about your illness / injury / disability?
- Where can you find answers? If trying Google, look first at reputable sources like the NHS.
- Are there any support groups you can join locally, on Facebook or elsewhere?

Is your illness / injury / disability likely to be permanent?

- Is the prognosis that you will "get better" at some point?
- Is the prognosis that you will get worse?
- Is your condition terminal?
- If you don't know this yet, when will you know (if at all)?
- What are your thoughts around this?
- Who can you talk to on this, to share the load?

Why this illness / injury / disability?

- Why this? Why this ailment? Why is this part of your body giving in, trying to get your attention? What's the relevance of your headache? What is the relevance of your heart problem, of your back pain, of your disability? What is it trying to tell you?
- The area of the body often correlates to what was happening for you in life and will help you work out the connection. If the connection is not becoming clear, talk it out with somebody else, and that often helps you to find clarity.

Why is it happening now?

- Why now? Why is this experience happening at this moment in time? Why wasn't it two weeks ago? Why wasn't it two years ago?
- What is the message that your body wants you to get in this moment?
- Start to think of these signals as friendly, like your internal fire alarm is trying to alert you. It's trying to say, "Um, there's smoke here. I just want to give you a heads-up."

What signs were there beforehand?

- What signs might you have missed? A lot of times, we think that an ailment has hit us suddenly. This can happen with certain conditions, but the body usually starts to give subtle signals beforehand – and if you're not listening to your body, it progresses and worsens until you find yourself in bed, calling in sick to work, wondering how this all happened.
- How early did you pick up any signs and signals?

What other areas need to be healed?

- What else needs to be healed? The body often reflects the pain, suffering, miscommunication, disconnection, and imbalances in somebody's external life. The physical world is not separate from your mental, emotional, social and spiritual arenas. They arere all connected.
- Where is it that you feel out of balance, and how might other areas of your life also be connected to your condition?

What would you like to say about it all?

- If you spoke from the heart, what would you say about having become ill / acquiring your disability?
- This is probably the most powerful question, giving permission to say what is in deep inside you, or even what you have been keeping hidden from yourself.
- Are you afraid? Are you secretly glad to have to take time off and take stock? Are you depressed / worried about not regaining your full health again?.

How does the illness / injury / disability affect your home life?

- What effect(s) do you have from your condition which make your home life difficult?
- What was your physical health like beforehand, what was your mental health situation, were you under stress and strain in personal life or at work?
- Can you manage your daily living alongside your illness / injury / disability?
- Can you see a way through this?

Is your illness / injury / disability related to drug or alcohol dependency?

It is known that trauma is a major source for addiction or problematic alcohol/drug use. What that trauma is, is very personal to each individual. It could come through the form of ill health when all of a sudden life changes.

You might feel a sense grief for the loss of your old self and what that old self used to be able to do.

This could include feeling frustrated at not being able to carry out your job to the best of your ability, unable to concentrate for long periods, or physically unable to sit or stand long enough to do your job.

It is important to note that you don't have to be physically dependant on a substance / alcohol in order to have an issue that needs addressing.

Using a substance or alcohol may have started out as a way to cope with feelings or illness that you felt unable to deal with in any other way.

Realising you have a problem with drugs or alcohol is the first step to getting better, but it's often the hardest one. Look for as much support as you can to help you with this.

- Have you spoken with your doctor?
- Do you have support within your home / family / friends?

There are many services offering support for substance or alcohol dependency – please contact the one in your local area.

On the next two pages there are two series of questions to determine a person's alcohol dependency.

The units referred to are:

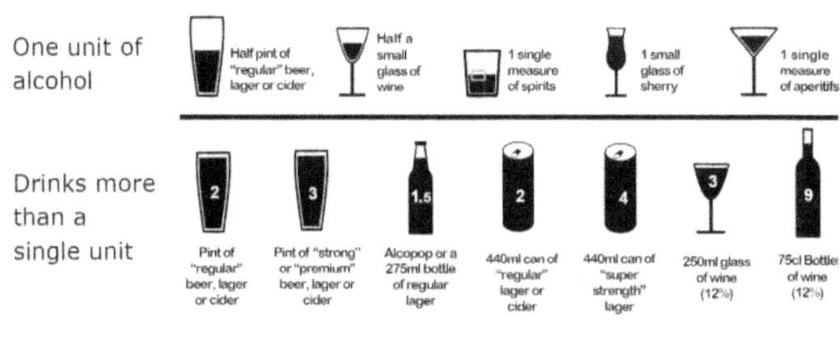

Fast alcohol screening test (FAST)

FAST is an alcohol harm assessment tool. It consists of a subset of questions from the full alcohol use disorders identification test (**AUDIT**).

FAST was developed for use in emergency departments, but can be used in a variety of health and social care settings.

Questions	Scoring system				
	0	**1**	**2**	**3**	**4**
How often have you had 6 or more units if female, or 8 or more if male, on a single occasion in the last year?	Never	Less than monthly	Monthly	Weekly	Daily or almost daily
Only answer the following questions if the answer above is Never (0), Less than monthly (1) or Monthly (2). **Stop here if your answer is Weekly (3) or Daily (4).**					
How often during the last year have you failed to do what was normally expected from you because of your drinking?	Never	Less than monthly	Monthly	Weekly	Daily or almost daily
How often during the last year have you been unable to remember what happened the night before because you had been drinking?	Never	Less than monthly	Monthly	Weekly	Daily or almost daily
Has a relative or friend, doctor or other health worker been concerned about your drinking or suggested that you cut down?	No		Yes, but not in the last year		Yes, during the last year
Add up your total FAST score: **3 or more** on the first question, or on all 4 questions is a FAST positive result.					

If your score is **FAST positive**, complete the remaining **AUDIT** alcohol screening questions; this may include the three remaining questions above as well as the six questions below to obtain a full AUDIT score.

Questions	Scoring system				
	0	1	2	3	4
How often do you have a drink containing alcohol?	Never	Monthly or less	2 to 4 times per month	2 to 3 times per week	4 times or more per week
How many units of alcohol do you drink on a typical day when you are drinking?	0 to 2	3 to 4	5 to 6	7 to 8	10 or more
How often during the last year have you found that you were not able to stop drinking once you had started?	Never	Less than monthly	Monthly	Weekly	Daily or almost daily
How often during the last year have you needed an alcoholic drink in the morning to get yourself going after a heavy drinking session?	Never	Less than monthly	Monthly	Weekly	Daily or almost daily
How often during the last year have you had a feeling of guilt or remorse after drinking?	Never	Less than monthly	Monthly	Weekly	Daily or almost daily
Have you or somebody else been injured as a result of your drinking?	No		Yes, but not in the last year		Yes, during the last year

Add up your total AUDIT score:

    0 to 7 indicates low risk

    8 to 15 indicates increasing risk

    16 to 19 indicates higher risk,

    20 or more indicates possible dependence.

How (and when) do you decide that you are ill enough to see a doctor?

- How long have you been ill / sick?
- How ill / incapacitated do you feel you need to be to warrant seeing a doctor? This book is going to press during the Covid19 pandemic – you may be avoiding doctors' surgeries, hospitals or clinics because of this.
- Could you talk with a pharmacist / helpline?
- Can you schedule to see a doctor before or after your work schedule?
- If the only available times are during your normal working hours, how easy / difficult would it be for you to attend?

SPACE FOR EXTRA NOTES

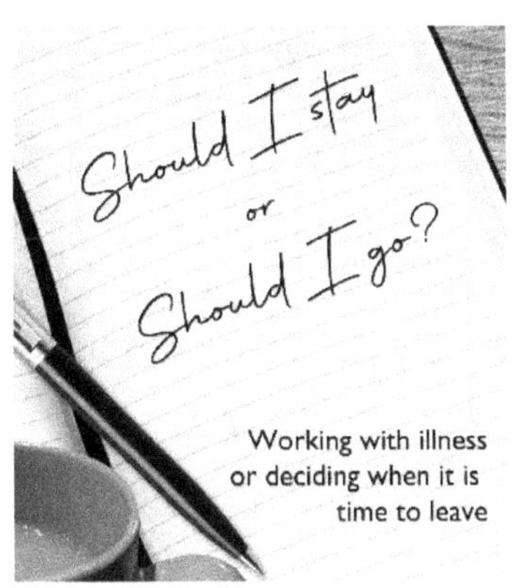

How well are you dealing with your condition?

How well are you PHYSICALLY coping with your condition?

- On a scale of zero ("not at all, I can't cope") to ten ("I can manage very well"), how well are you physically dealing with your illness / injury / disability?
- How well are you coping at home?
- How well are you coping at work?
- How well are you dealing with any medications / treatments / medical appointments?

How well are you MENTALLY coping with your condition?

- On a scale of zero ("not at all, I can't cope") to ten ("I can manage very well"), how well are you mentally coping with your illness / injury / disability?
- How well are you coping at home?
- How well are you coping at work?
- How well are you coping with having to take required medications / treatments / attend medical appointments?

> **What is your own attitude towards your illness / injury / disability?**

- Are you fighting against recognising that you are ill?
- Do you feel ashamed of it?
- Do you hate it / want to reject the diagnosis?
- Do you accept it / are you resigned to it? (Note: there's a difference!)

> **Is your illness / injury / disability visible or invisible?**

- A broken leg can be seen and immediately understood – even empathised with – by others. A bad back or constant migraines can be less easily understood, and depression even less.
- Is your condition visible or invisible?
- What difference does this make to you?
- Do you yourself feel visible or invisible as a result of your illness / injury / disability?
- Do you feel ignored, belittled, badly treated or pushed to one side? Who by?

Is your condition difficult for you to talk about?

- It can be particularly hard to discuss mental health issues or gynaecological problems with a male boss, or you might not have anyone who you feel understands.
- Is your condition something that you feel comfortable discussing with your doctor?
- Or your family / friends /?
- Or your employer?
- Or your colleagues?
- Do you know anyone else who has had this condition who you could talk with about their experience?

> **Some thoughts on caring for someone else – it might not actually be YOU who is ill / disabled / injured. You might be needing time off to care for someone else.**

Your job:

- What provision is there (if any) in your work contract for this situation?
- How long can you take time off to care for someone else?
- Will you get paid during this time off – and can you manage financially during it?
- Can you take time out in your working day to take the person you are caring for to medical appointments?
- What level of support do you get from your workplace?

The person you are looking after:

- What support is there for the person you are looking after – mentally, physically, financially?
- How well are they coping with the situation?
- Is the person you are caring for receiving the correct level of financial support / benefits to be able to cope with their illness? Check this with your local council or Social Care team.
- Can your local Social Care team provide carers to assist with physical care?
- Can the ill person afford this assistance, or any other private carer?

Who supports the carer?

- What support is there for you as a carer – mentally, physically, financially?
- How well are you coping with the situation?
- Are you the sole person taking care of someone who is ill?
- Where can you get support from? Check with your local Social Care team.

If you are experiencing mental stress or strain related to your illness, injury or disability, what can help you?

- Alongside a physical illness / injury / disability you will probably also be experiencing some level of mental stress / strain as your condition progresses.
- You could be suffering from workplace stress, dealing with a relationship breakdown, going through grief or loss – or you may have a mental health disorder / illness.
- Before becoming ill, how was your mental health - and how is it now?
- Do you know what kind of help / support you need?
- Do you need time / help to come to terms with your condition?
- Are those around you able to support you?
- Have you considered therapy to help you?

(Further information is in the Accessing Appropriate Mental Health Support section.)

SPACE FOR EXTRA NOTES

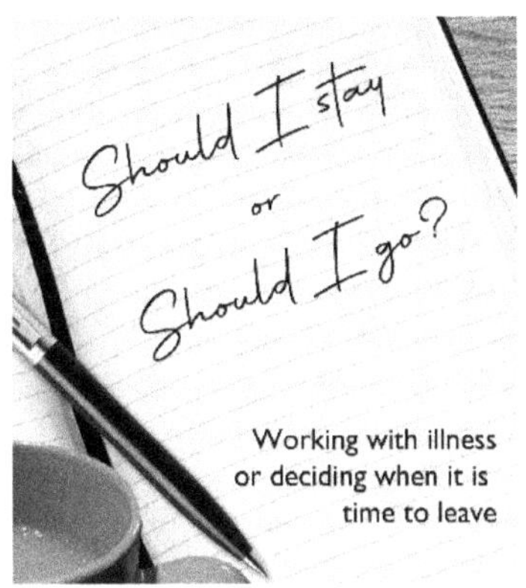

How is your ability to work affected?

How does the illness / injury / disability affect your ability to do your job?

- What effect(s) do you have from your condition which impact on your working?
- Are you able to concentrate enough to carry out your work?
- Are you able to sit / stand / move about appropriately to continue working?
- Does any medication / treatment impair your ability to work?
- To continue working, would you need to make any adaptations to your workspace – e.g. a different chair, desk, computer aids?

When should you continue to work and when should you take time off?

- Do you feel that your illness / injury / disability is manageable enough for you to continue working?
- Is this sustainable in the long term?
- How much does your condition affect your general wellbeing?
- Are you feeling stressed from your condition?
- Would you be better to take some time off in order to then return to work afresh?

What is your employer's attitude towards your illness / injury / disability?

- Do you feel that your condition is understood by your employer?
- Are they acting negatively or positively towards you?
- How do you feel about this?
- Do you feel that they understand how it affects you?
- Could you send them some information about the condition, to help them understand better?

If you need to take time off, what is detailed in your organisation's absence policy?

- What is permitted for attending doctor's appointments?
- What is the procedure for taking time off?
- Has your doctor given you a Fitness for Work certificate (previously known as a sick note)?
- Are you entitled to sick leave – whether on full pay, half pay, no pay or anything in between – and for how long on each of these?

If you are on sick leave, when can / should you make yourself available by phone / email / video call from home?

- How necessary would it be for someone at your organisation to reach you while you take time off?
- Could someone else take up the more vital elements of your role?
- Think carefully before you offer to be available by phone / email / video – does this go against your company's sickness policy / working time regs / your doctor's recommendations / your health needs?

Future planning in your job - creating a procedural folder

- If you haven't already done this, something you should think about for the future is to create a folder containing details of the most essential elements of your role. This would be useful not just for covering while you are taking time off for your illness / injury / disability, but will help in succession planning for whenever you leave or retire.
- Use the space below to list the vital elements of your job for which you could create instructions.

> **Taking yourself seriously – both about your role and your health**

- No one wants a sick employee coughing in the office, and spreading their germs. Some people though fear taking sick leave. This can lead to 'presenteeism', which can create further issues – either the illness being spread or shared, or higher absence as the person becomes worse, leading to more time off.
- Do you feel pressurised to stay at work, or to return to work, while you are ill?
- Your health needs to last you for your whole lifetime. How much care are you taking of it?

Has your illness gone on for a long time and you need further medical intervention / additional time off?

- Is your illness getting worse with time?
- When / how often should you return to your doctor?
- When should you push for a referral to a specialist or a clinic?
- How long have you been ill / disabled?
- How long has your ability to work been affected?
- Are you coming to the end of your sick leave entitlement?
- Are your employers looking for a second medical opinion?
- When should you / can you return to work?

Some additional thinking points on taking time off from work.

Have you thought about any of the following?

- "I was off work all week and on Saturday I dragged myself out to do some urgent food shopping. I saw and spoke to a colleague. I'm worried they will think I was faking it because I was at the supermarket."
- "I posted a photo on Facebook in my garden, now my colleagues say I wasn't ill."
- "One of my colleagues keeps calling me, even though I'm supposed to off work. I need to tell them to stop disturbing me while I am ill."
- "But they need me, I'm indispensable!" – really? Who else could help them in your absence?
- How did the company manage without you before you started working there?
- Remember – if you died tomorrow, the organisation would replace your role or pass the work to someone else within a relatively short time.
- What technology / systems / ideas do you have which would help your boss to continue without you while you concentrate on your health?
- "How much should I tell my colleagues about my illness?"
- You do not need to justify your time off to colleagues, nor do they need to know any details unless you wish to share them.

Some thinking points on reactions from your boss and colleagues who don't seem to take your illness / injury / disability seriously.

- "My boss doesn't think I'm THAT ill".
- If you doctor says take time off work, you should. It's not macho or 'strong' to flog yourself. What could you say to your boss to make them think seriously about your condition?
- A colleague saying to you "So-and-so had the same issue but they came to work" – so the unasked question is "why can't you?"
- The trouble with so many chronic illnesses is that most people won't want to believe you when you say to them that you are too ill to work.
- They will tell you that you look great, that it might be in your head only, that it is likely stress, that everything will be okay.
- Alternatively they may offer unqualified advice, suggesting inappropriate treatments or ways of making yourself feel better.
- None of these are the right things to say to someone whose entire existence is a fairly consistent torture of the body and mind.
- People might say these things because they are well-intentioned usually, because they wish you the best, but they also say it because you make them uncomfortable.
- This is because your presence and your illness is evidence of the fact that each and every one of us is able to become ill, so ill that we are not able to continue with our daily lives – and that is hard for them to accept.

SPACE FOR EXTRA NOTES

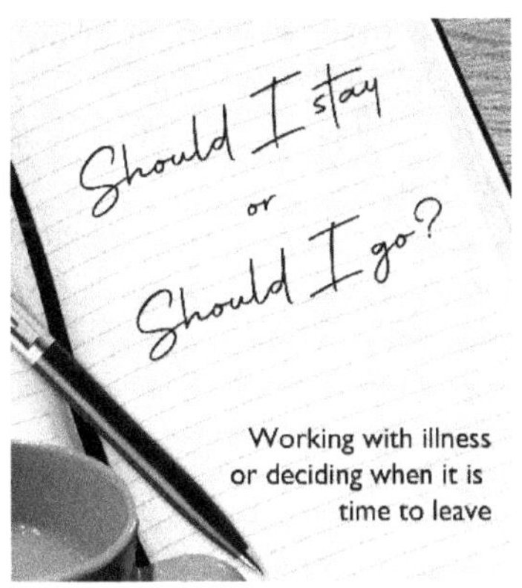

Is your condition a result of your job?

Is your health condition a direct or indirect result of your job?

- Many health issues can be work related. Have you experienced any of the following?
- Workplace accident, poor working conditions or practices, bad health and safety, back / posture / joint problems from poor equipment, faulty lighting causing migraines, mental health problems from stress and strain or a change of management structure where you no longer fit, injured in an incident with colleagues or customers, working with dangerous substances?
- Can you see a direct connection between your condition and your job?

Is your health issue related to being stressed by your workload?

- Are you stressed because you have to meet impossible targets, there's too much work for one person to ever complete, or feel there's no light at the end of the tunnel?
- Have you been made to feel inadequate, not good enough, a burden, a loser?
- Have you kept a diary of your workload?
- Have you contacted your Human Resources team and/or someone in management?
- Contact your union representative to discuss this with them.

Is your health issue related to your working relationship with a colleague or your boss?

- If your condition relates to a staffing issue, it can be very difficult to insist on any changes being made.
- Have you kept a diary to log any incidents?
- If not, can you backtrack to create an accurate representation of events?
- Do you have any witnesses or evidence relating to what happened?
- Contact your Human Resources department.
- Contact your union representative to discuss this with them.

Have you experienced sexual harassment, bullying, verbal / physical abuse in the workplace?

- Some workplaces have a distinctly "macho" culture, where staff have to act tough and work in gruelling circumstances. There are also managers who have no idea how to manage people. And there are downright bullies, who haven't moved on from their playground antics from childhood.
- Have you been bullied at work?
- Has this led to you being unwell?
- Have other staff left because they felt unsupported?
- Do you feel you are supported?
- Contact your union representative to discuss this with them.

Some thoughts on accidents / illnesses which are related to your job / workplace.

According to UK trade unions over 2.5m people are made ill by their job every year, with more than 28 million working days lost due to sickness caused or made worse by work.

Whatever the symptoms or causes of workplace sickness, you have the legal right to be kept safe and healthy by employers and should never have to work with equipment or substances that could endanger your health. Everything from serious accidents to poor lifting techniques can have an adverse impact on your health

Many of the factors that cause workplace illnesses are avoidable by following proper safety rules and carrying out regular Risk Assessments.

Bad working practices and poor health and safety measures are usually to blame for workplace illnesses, even though your employer has a legal duty to keep you safe.

Some of the most common work related illness in the UK are :

- Asthma
- Back pain
- Cognitive disfunction
- Musculo skeletal disorders
- Gastro-intestinal problems
- Noise damage
- Psychiatric conditions
- Skin diseases
- Stress related illnesses – anxiety or depression
- Unintended weight loss or gain
- Vibrating injuries
- Vocal injuries
- Weakened immune system.

UK health and safety law is extensive and covers almost every possible factor that could make you ill or the victim of an accident.

The UK Health and Safety Commission and the Health and Safety Executive are responsible for creating and enforcing safety laws.

If you feel you have been made ill or are facing unacceptable risks at work check with the HSE.

Failure to comply with health and safety law is a serious offence.

All workers have statutory rights around health and safety so your employer cannot take any action against you for reporting problems.

Trade unions also have the legal right to investigate health risks on your behalf.

Many workplaces have union safety representatives so you should always ask for help if you feel that your job is putting you at risk.

Accidents at work

If you have had an accident at work, you should ensure that the accident is appropriately recorded by reporting it at work and seeing a doctor.

It's also a good idea to:

- make notes about your accident as soon as possible - you can include drawings if they'll help show what happened
- take photographs of your injury and whatever caused your accident
- make sure you have contact details for anyone who witnessed your accident
- ask any witnesses to make notes and share them with you.

Reporting accidents

Who you report your accident to depends on:

- where you were working when you had it
- your 'employment status' - this means whether you're an employee, a worker or self-employed

Seeing a doctor

Make an appointment to see your GP as soon as possible.

They can record the details of your accident in your medical records, as well as treat your injury.

Ask them to refer you to a specialist as soon as possible, if necessary – contesting any workplace injury or illness can be a lengthy process and there are usually maximum legal timescales involved.

If you have already become ill your doctor can issue a sick note and provide advice on the cause of your condition and any rehabilitation required to improve it.

Check your contract of employment to see if:

- your employer has to give you paid time off for your appointment
- you are eligible for 'contractual sick pay, or
- you have access to an employee assistance helpline or medical care.

What should you do if you want to make a compensation claim?

You might want to claim for your injury if it was your employer's or client's fault. Contact Citizens Advice for help finding a specialist solicitor, or contact your local union representative – they will help you decide what to do and could attend meetings with your employer to support you.

Either way, get legal advice as soon as possible if you want to make a claim, because there are time limits, and it is a complex area of law.

- You may have experienced a difficult time at work and you may be left with a related illness – but that does not necessarily mean you will be able to make a claim..
- If your illness is from workplace stress, compensation claim can only be brought in more extreme cases of a recognised psychiatric illness such as clinical depression.
- Any claim will need to show that your condition was caused by your workplace or your job –a specialist's report will probably be needed.
- You need evidence that the employer was at fault – they not only 'exposed' you to the situation but knew (or should have predicted) that this could lead to your illness.
- You will need to show that your employer was specifically made aware of the problems you were facing at work – e.g. that you were not coping with the volume or type of work
- Finally, having shown that your employer knew of your situation your lawyers will need to be able to show that they failed to adequately help you.

SPACE FOR EXTRA NOTES

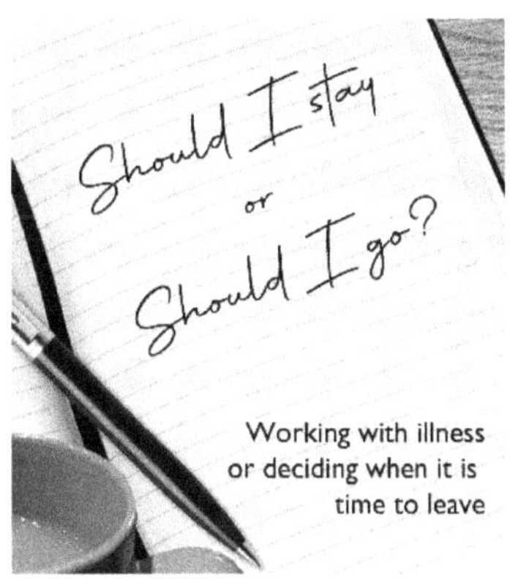

What could help you continue in your job?

Do you need to continue your job by working from home, or perhaps work shorter hours?

- Do you know your rights on requesting flexible working? Check with the Citizens' Advice Bureau.
- With many of us working from home during the Covid19 pandemic, you may already be doing this – is it sustainable for you?
- If you are not already working from home, could you request this?
- Would shorter / different working hours help you to manage your condition better?

Are there some changes that could be made relatively easily at your job which would make it easier for you to stay?

- Would a different type of chair help you?
- Or a different desk – standing desks are available.
- Could your working space be rearranged if it is too bright, too dark, too hot, too cold, too far from the toilet facilities?
- Does your building have a lift for you to get upstairs?
- Could you move to another area in the premises that is better suited to you?
- Could you learn / adapt to different ways of working to take your new condition into account?

Are there some more difficult / controversial / expensive changes that could make it easier for you to stay in your role?

- Do you need special toileting, changing or rest facilities?
- Do you need a designated space for taking medications (e.g. injections) at work?
- Your mobility may be affected by your condition – do you need a ramp to enable you to access the building?
- Can you physically get around within the building? Are doorways wide enough for a wheelchair, for example?
- Would you need some colleagues to undergo some form of training in what to do to help you if you have a seizure at work, if you need help taking your medications, if you need assistance to get around the building?

What is your workplace's culture around health issues - is it a macho "you must work at 100% level until you are dead" or healthy place?

- Is being home on sick leave frowned upon in your company's culture?
- Do you and your colleagues dread being ill and having to take time off because of the repercussions?
- On the upside, does your company provide access to any healthcare facilities that could help you – a gym, a pool, a spa, a fitness centre?

What are your role's sickness conditions? (Not just how much time you are entitled to.)

What are the conditions regarding:
- pay during time off,
- how much time off is permitted,
- what form of medical notes / self certification the company requires,
- sick leave interviews, questions, home visits,
- urging you to return quickly,
- pressures to return,
- threats to your role's continuance or of procedures being instigated against you,
- back to work interviews?

Do you need to stay in your job in order to access your current and/or future healthcare?

Some further thoughts on what you might need in order to continue in your current job.

This is not just a question of what physical aids you might need to continue in your role.

Aspects to consider are:

- Can you contractually stay in your job – can you still fulfil the requirements of your contract of employment?
- Can you physically stay – can you physically manage to do the work and can you do it for the same hours?
- Can you mentally stay – can you manage to continue working and maintain good mental health whilst doing so?
- Can you financially stay – if you have to change your role or hours of working, can you manage on whatever rate of pay you might have to change to?
- Can you stay in terms of medical care – can you manage your medications and medical appointments without infringing too much on your work?
- Can you adapt to needing physical aides in order to continue working? – and can your organisation adapt in order to allow this?
- Can you see yourself learning new ways to carry out your work, in order to adapt to your new physical / mental condition?
- Can you deal with the attitudes / reactions of those around you – can you cope with how colleagues might treat you for example if you have a terminal illness or have had to undergo surgery which has changed you physically?
- Can you manage your illness alongside your home life, and still have time / energy / motivation enough to continue with your job?
- How would you cope physically, mentally and financially if your company asks /or tells you to leave / terminates your contract?

SPACE FOR EXTRA NOTES

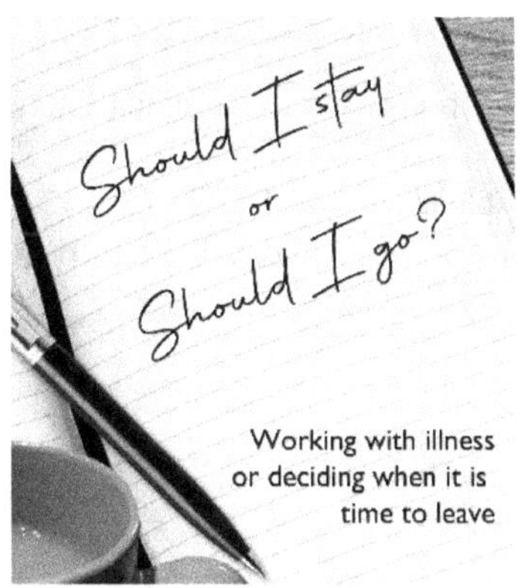

What do you need / want?

What help do you need?

- What are you immediate physical and mental needs?
- Do you need assistance in your daily living – be it medical aids or a person to do something for you?
- Are you physically mobile? Can you get around the house or outside?
- Do you need to order your shopping online as you can't get out?
- Are you unable to physically get to work?
- How may any of these change in the future?

Do you need changes made to your home to adapt to your condition, and are there funds you can apply to for help with this?

- In the UK, you should check with your local council's Adult Social Care department to see if they can assist. They can provide medical aids for use in and around the home.
- Depending on your illness, injury or disability, there may be a private trust which could offer some support.
- Check Facebook groups for details of any further support options.

Is your illness something that you need to inform other bodies about?

- For example, in the UK if your eyesight has been affected by your illness / injury . disability, you have experienced a stroke or you have been diagnosed with Obstructive Sleep Apnoea, there are legal requirements that you must inform your Driving Licence authority.
- Check with your doctors and any support group related to your condition.

How much do you NEED this job?

- Answer this question in terms of:
- Needing the money
- Wanting personal satisfaction
- Needing something to challenge you
- Need for maintaining a routine
- Not wanting to feel you are "giving in"
- Needing something to do / time filler
- Needing a sense of continuity despite difficult circumstances
- Needing to feel useful / purposeful...

How much do you WANT this job?

(There's a difference between wanting THIS job and wanting ANY job...)

- Do you want THIS job, or just any job?
- How important to you is what you actually do at work?
- Are you clutching at straws to maintain a sense of normality?
- Would you prefer to be doing something else?
- Have you been wanting a change, but not made any plans to do it? Is now the time to think about it more?

SPACE FOR EXTRA NOTES

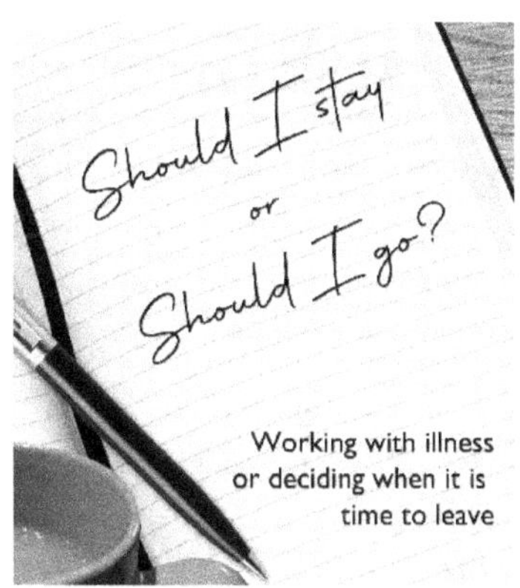

Information on accessing appropriate mental health support

The importance of seeking support in our mental health – particularly during the Covid19 pandemic.

MIND, the UK mental health charity reported in October 2020:

"World Mental Health Day 2020 is the most important one yet. This year has been a tough one for us all. The months of lockdown and loss have had a huge impact on our mental health.

According to our research, with over 16,000 people, we know that more than half of adults (60%) and over two thirds of young people (68%) said their mental health got worse during lockdown.

We know that many have developed new mental health problems as a result of the pandemic and, for some of us, existing mental health problems have gotten worse."

Good stress management is important in the workplace.

If you often experience feelings of stress, you might be at risk of developing a mental health problem, like depression or anxiety, and stress can also make existing problems worse. Building resilience can help you to adapt to challenging circumstances.

You don't need to cope with stress alone. Here are some general things you can try:

- Recognising the signs of stress and the causes is a good place to start.
- Work out what you find stressful and helpful in the workplace. Once you know what works for you, talk to your employer about this. They may be able to make some changes to help you.
- Try different coping techniques to use as soon as you start to feel pressure building. Everyone is different, so it may take time to find a method that works for you.
- Try mindfulness. Focusing on the here and now can help you to create space to respond in new ways to situations.
- Look after your physical health - physical activity and food and can help your mental health.
- Ask for help. Everyone needs a hand from time to time. If you are over-worked, discuss your workload with your manager – you need to talk with them about setting more realistic

targets and how you can solve any problems that you're having.

- Balance your time - don't do too much at once.
- Reward yourself for achievements.
- Be realistic. You don't have to be 'perfect' all the time.
- Make a Wellness Action Plan to map out what causes you stress and what keeps you well at work. Make use of other support already on offer. Some organisations provide employee assistance programmes (EAPs) which give free advice and counselling. Others have internal systems such as mentoring or buddy systems.
- If you don't feel supported, communicate this. If you feel you can't talk to your boss, speak or write to your human resources department or trade union representative if you have one.
- Work hard to develop good relationships with your colleagues. Connecting with them can help to build up a network of support and make being at work more enjoyable. They can also have your back when you are experiencing difficulties."

You may not consider yourself to be suffering from mental health difficulties while you are dealing with your illness, disability or injury – but continued time off work, medical appointments, treatments, and worries about whether you can remain in your job or how you are going to make ends meet at the end of the month can all have a negative affect on your mental health. It can feel bad enough to be ill – but to have sleepless nights due to worrying about being ill can make things worse.

Talking through your fears, worries and how your illness affects you can be incredibly helpful – especially with a trained therapist. Within the next few pages there is some information on how therapy could help you.

Some points on how counselling or psychotherapy could help you.

Before the start of the COVID-19 pandemic, it was estimated that 1 in 4 people were struggling with a mental health issue.

No doubt this will have increased as people now have all the issues they had before the pandemic plus they have developed new issues around anxiety, financial hardship, changing relationships, dealing with isolation and loneliness, overwhelm, burnout, loss and bereavement.

In addition, people who weren't struggling with a mental health issue before the pandemic are now struggling too.

Seeing a counsellor isn't just about dealing with your mental health, it's also for those who have all manner of life issues.

You might be referred for counselling via your doctor's surgery, or they can point you towards a service to which you can self-refer.

You may also see advertisements for counsellors and therapists in health related magazines and websites, plus you can search via Google for "counselling near me".

There should be no stigma about seeing a therapist to talk through your problem.

What is the difference between 'counselling' and 'psychotherapy'?
Counselling usually refers to a brief treatment that centres around behaviour patterns.
A counsellor generally puts their focus to what's happening to you in the present.
This could be difficulties at work/home, one specific traumatic event such as a bad break up or losing your job, or even just feeling more stressed than usual.
The counsellor will look at your immediate presenting symptoms and behaviour (e.g. feeling more anxious than usual) and how

that's impacting your life. They will focus on equipping you with workable, short-term tools that can help you break out of negative thoughts and habits.

Psychotherapy focuses on working with clients for a longer-term and draws from insight into emotional problems and difficulties – and is more in-depth. The psychotherapist will turn their focus to emotions and experiences you encountered growing up - as a child or young adult - as well as your presenting symptoms and issues, in order to shed light on how these experiences have shaped who you are today.

They will place an emphasis on creating a space for you to feel comfortable to open up and share experiences from your past. The idea being that once these buried experiences (and their accompanying emotions) are brought to the surface, they can be fully processed, and ultimately, released.

Whilst a counsellor might be more focused on helping you with symptoms (anxiety, stress, difficulties sleeping etc.), a psychotherapist also deals with mental health conditions that have developed over a longer period of time. This means a psychotherapist will work with more complex mental health conditions too, such as PTSD, OCD, and long-term anxiety disorders.

A registered / licensed psychotherapist will have also undergone a higher level of training than a counsellor – in the UK this is usually a Masters level degree.

Two clinical questionnaires that can help you determine if you can refer yourself to counselling or if you need to see a doctor.

The UK's national standard measures routinely used by doctors, therapists and psychiatrists as screening tools are the **GAD-7** for Anxiety and the **PHQ-9** for Depression.

Your scorings for each indicate how severe the issue is and whether you need to think about seeking help with your mental health.

For each question, write your score:

0 if your answer is 'not at all', 1 if 'several days', 2 if 'more than half the days' and 3 if 'nearly every day'.

GAD-7   Over the last two weeks how often have you been bothered by the following problems?

Feeling nervous, anxious, or on edge   ______
Not being able to stop or control worrying   ______
Worrying too much about different things   ______
Trouble relaxing   ______
Being so restless that it's hard to sit still   ______
Becoming easily annoyed or irritable   ______
Feeling afraid as if something awful might happen.

Your score total ______

Severity: None = 0 – 5   Mild = 6 - 10
                    Moderate = 11 - 15   Severe = 16 – 21

If you checked off any problems, how difficult have these problems made it for you to do your work, take care of things at home, or get along with other people?
Not difficult at all   ______
Somewhat difficult   ______
Very difficult   ______
Extremely difficult   ______

PHQ-9 **Over the last two weeks how often have you been bothered by the following problems?**	
Little interest or pleasure in doing things	____
Feeling down, depressed, or hopeless	____
Trouble falling or staying asleep, sleeping too much	____
Feeling tired or having little energy	____
Poor appetite or overeating	____
Feeling bad about yourself – or that you are a failure or have let yourself or your family down	____
Trouble concentrating on things, such as reading the newspaper or watching television	____
Moving or speaking so slowly that other people could have noticed. Or the opposite – being so fidgety or restless that you have been moving around a lot more than usual	____
Thoughts that you would be better off dead or of hurting yourself in some way	

Your score total ____

Severity: None = 0 – 4   Mild = 5 - 9
               Moderate = 10 - 14   Mod.Severe 15 - 19
               Severe = 20 – 27

If you checked off any problems, how difficult have these problems made it for you to do your work, take care of things at home or get along with other people?

Not difficult at all   ____
Somewhat difficult   ____
Very difficult   ____
Extremely difficult   ____

Please remember that both the GAD-7 and PHQ-9 tests are intended as tools to assist clinicians with identifying and diagnosing anxiety and depression but they are not a substitute for diagnosis by a trained clinician.

(source: Spitzer, R. L., Kroenke, K., Williams, J. B. W., & Lowe, B. (2006). A brief measure for assessing generalized anxiety disorder - The GAD-7. Archives of Internal Medicine, 166, 1092-1097)

What can you expect to happen if you go to see a counsellor or psychotherapist?

(reproduced from https://psychcentral.com/lib/what-to-expect-in-your-first-counseling-session)

Are you about to go to a counsellor or psychotherapist for the first time? Whatever your reason for seeking help, you will be more at ease and get better results if you know what to expect.

In your first session, the therapist typically will ask certain questions about you and your life. This information helps them make an initial assessment of your situation.

Questions they might ask include:
- Why you sought therapy. A particular issue probably led you to seek counselling. The therapist has to understand your surface problem(s) before he can get to the deeper issues.
- Your personal history and current situation. The therapist will ask you a series of questions about your life. For example, because family situations play an important role in who you are, they will ask about your family history and your current family situation.
- Your current symptoms. Other than knowing the reason you sought therapy, the therapist will attempt to find out if you're suffering from other symptoms of your problem. For example, your problem might be causing difficulty at work.

The therapist will use this information to better understand your problem. And, while they may make a diagnosis at the end of your first visit, it's more likely that a diagnosis will take a few more sessions.

Don't just sit there. Therapy is a team effort. If you don't take an active part in the session, you won't find the counselling experience valuable. Here are some things you can do to make your first session as successful as possible.

Be open. Therapists are trained to ask the right questions, but they're not mind readers. The therapist can do his job more effectively if you answer the questions openly and honestly.

Be prepared. Before you get to the session, know how to describe "what's wrong," and to describe your feelings about your problem. One way to prepare is to write down the reasons you're seeking help. Make a list and then read it out loud. Hearing yourself say it a few times will help you describe things more clearly to the therapist.

Ask questions. The more you understand how counselling works, the more comfortable you'll be, so ask questions about the process, and ask the therapist to repeat anything you don't understand.

Be open and honest about your feelings. A lot will be going through your head in this first session. Listen to your own reactions and feelings, and share them with the therapist. You'll both learn from these insights.

Be sure to go to your first session with realistic expectations.

Therapy is not a quick fix for your problem, rather it is a process. With some effort on your part and a strong relationship with your therapist, it can be a successful tool toward resolving problems.

You may be referred to your local EA in IAPT service for help:

About IAPT

At the time of publication (January 2021) only 32% of people with mental illness in the UK are in work, compared with 48% of people with a disability and 80% of people who do not have a disability

IAPT is the 'Improving Access to Psychological Therapies' programme of delivering talking therapies.

The 'Employment Advisors in IAPT' contract is an extension of a trial funded by the Department of Work and Pensions / National Health Service Joint Work and Health Unit, running in 40% of CCG areas in England. Since 2008, it has transformed the treatment of adult anxiety disorders and depression.

IAPT is widely-recognised as the most ambitious programme of talking therapies in the world and in the past year alone more than one million people accessed IAPT services for help to overcome their depression and anxiety, and better manage their mental health.

IAPT services are characterized by three things:

- Evidenced-based psychological therapies: with the therapy delivered by fully trained and accredited practitioners, matched to the mental health problem and its intensity and duration designed to optimize outcomes. From April 2018 all clinical commissioning groups are required to offer IAPT services integrated with physical healthcare pathways. The IAPT Pathway for People with Long-term Physical Health Conditions and Medically Unexplained Symptoms guidance is intended to help with implementation and sets out the ideal pathway for IAPT services.

- Routine outcome monitoring: so that the person having therapy and the clinician offering it have up-to-date information on an individual's progress. This supports the development of a positive and shared approach to the goals of therapy and as this data is anonymized and published this promotes transparency in service performance encouraging improvement.

- Regular and outcomes focused supervision so practitioners are supported to continuously improve and deliver high quality care.

The priorities for service development are:

- Expanding services so that 1.9m adults access treatment each year by 2024.
- Focusing on people with long term conditions. Two thirds of people with a common mental health problem also have a long term physical health problem, greatly increasing the cost of their care by an average of 45% more than those without a mental health problem. By integrating IAPT services with physical health services the NHS can provide better support to this group of people and achieve better outcomes.
- Supporting people to find or stay in work. Good work contributes to good mental health, and IAPT services can better contribute to improved employment outcomes.
- Improving quality and people's experience of services. Improving the numbers of people who recover, reducing geographic variation between services, and reducing inequalities in access and outcomes for particular population groups are all important aspects of the development of IAPT services.

The 'EA in IAPT' programme

'EA in IAPT' sees Employment Advisors working alongside Improving Access to Psychological Therapy clinicians, to allow employment support to be routinely offered to IAPT clients.

This increases the provision of combined mental health treatment and employment support, and standardises and improves the quality of employment support provided in IAPT services.

Employment Advisors support IAPT services to achieve better outcomes for clients and sustain these outcomes after they are discharged.

The contract makes a major contribution to the UK Government target to enable an extra 29,000 people with mental illness a year to receive employment support by 2021.

IAPT services around the UK ae run differently in each area – in Derbyshire, Employment Advisors provided by Ingeus work alongside clinicians within the county's IAPT providers.

Ally Campbell at Ingeus (Team Manager, EA in IAPT) writes:

"EA in IAPT is run across a number of CCGs in England. Most are employed within the IAPT provider, whereas two (Derbyshire and Surrey) are commissioned for their regions and are managed by an external employment support specialist company and are embedded within multiple providers.

"There is also some variation on length of support – some areas only work with clients whilst they are in IAPT and exit them at discharge, whereas in my area (Derbyshire) we work with the client until they achieve their outcome and/or are in a suitable place to agree exit.

"Since COVID-19 our delivery has been fully remote…. We have seen an increase in some topics (such as furlough, employee rights regarding health and safety, and redundancy) as well as complex cases (such as clients who experience bereavement or other life events alongside their therapy and employment support, and clients who have multiple and/or changing employment support needs – such as starting with us whilst in work and need supporting, to then face redundancy, have redundancy confirmed, and begin to job hunt, secure new work, and then receive in work support).

"We also have clients who are facing significant obstacles in their job search / job change goals, such as increased applicant numbers per vacancy (meaning also increased support neds for managing rejection and building resilience) and shifts in employment sectors and job roles available."

What the EA in IAPT programme can offer to you:
(For the terms of this programme, the therapist / counsellor is referred to as the 'clinician', and the person attending for help is the 'client'.)
When someone is referred to the programme, the process is:
The Clinician will identify, together with the client, the appropriate time to start work with an Employment Advisor.

The Employment Advisor will address work related issues or factors associated with returning back to employment, including the provision of information, advice and guidance around employment ranging from benefits, helping to resolve a conflict at work, helping to arrange reasonable adjustments in the workplace, signposting to other agencies, employer engagement, job search support, helping employers to make workplace adjustments or supporting them to understand the impact of health in the workplace, helping to practice interview skills and sourcing suitable job vacancies.

The clinician will address the client's emotional and mental wellbeing, including helping the advisor to address any issues associated with the client's mental health that is impacting on their employment e.g. the therapist will address the psychological blocks where this relates to work i.e. anxiety at interviews.

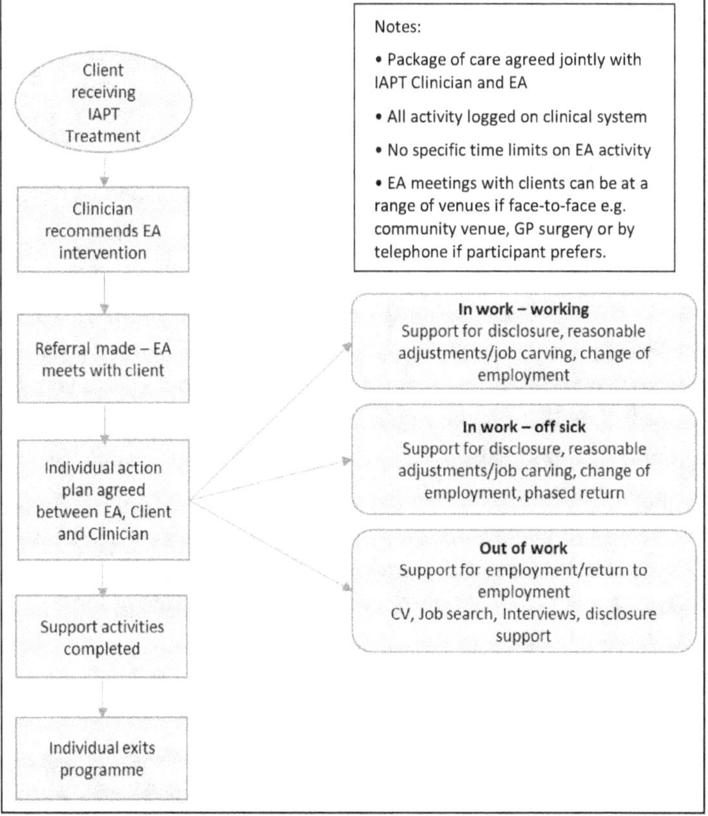

The often unspoken question – is your illness / disability / condition so bad that you are feeling suicidal or thinking of hurting yourself?

You might be feeling so upset, angry and in pain that you believe these feelings will never end. But it's important to remember that they cannot and will not last.

Like all feelings, these ones will pass.

It may be that you feel so unwell or so drained or so depressed that there may seem to be no answer to your health condition, other than to harm yourself. You may even be thinking about suicide.

There can be many causes of suicidal feelings. Sometimes it is linked to an existing mental health issue, but often there is an underlying cause such as a traumatic experience, personal, work, financial or health problems, or even a side effect of medication.

There are steps you can take right now to stop yourself from acting on your suicidal thoughts. Everyone is different, so it's about finding what works best for you.

MIND, the UK mental health charity say: If you feel unable to keep yourself safe, it's a mental health emergency.

What are suicidal feelings?

Suicide is the act of intentionally taking your own life. Suicidal feelings can mean having abstract thoughts about ending your life or feeling that people would be better off without you.

Or it can mean thinking about methods of suicide or making clear plans to take your own life.

If you are feeling suicidal, you might be scared or confused by your feelings, and find them overwhelming. But please know that you are not alone. Many people think about suicide at some point in their life.

What does it feel like to be suicidal?

Different people have different experiences of suicidal feelings. You might feel unable to cope with the difficult feelings you are experiencing. You may feel less like you want to die and more like you cannot go on living the life you have.

These feelings may build over time or might change from moment to moment. And it's common to not understand why you feel this way.

How you might think or feel

- hopeless, like there is no point in living
- tearful and overwhelmed by negative thoughts
- unbearable pain that you can't imagine ending
- useless, not wanted or not needed by others
- desperate, as if you have no other choice
- like everyone would be better off without you
- cut off from your body or physically numb
- fascinated by death.

What you may experience

- poor sleep, including waking up earlier than you want to
- a change in appetite, weight gain or loss
- no desire to take care of yourself, for example neglecting your physical appearance
- wanting to avoid others
- making a will or giving away possessions
- struggling to communicate
- self-loathing and low self-esteem
- urges to self-harm.

Self-harming

Many people who self-harm don't want to kill themselves. Self-harming can be a kind of "survival strategy", providing a person with a way of coping with overwhelming emotions. However, self-harming is usually a sign that a person needs immediate help and support.

How long will I feel suicidal?

How long suicidal feelings last is different for everyone.

It is common to feel as if you'll never be happy or hopeful again.

With appropriate treatment and support, including self-care, the majority of people who have felt suicidal continue onwards to live fulfilling lives.

The earlier you let someone know how you're feeling, the quicker you'll be able to get support to overcome these feelings - but it can feel difficult to open up to people.

Suicide due to workplace stress / illness

Suicidal thoughts can often be linked to issues such as workplace stress, bullying or harassment.

Every year between 5,500 and 6,000 people in the UK end their own lives – well over three times the number of people who die on our roads.

Unions can have a role to play in helping prevent suicides and supporting those who may have suicidal thoughts.

There are two main areas where union representatives can help make it less likely that someone in their workplace will end their lives:

- **Prevention**

  Unions can try to ensure that the workplace is not contributing to your mental health problems by tackling issues such as stress, bullying and harassment.

  They can also ensure that your employer has processes in place to help identify individuals at risk, support those people and raise awareness of the complex issues surrounding suicide.

  The union's role can include negotiating policies that cover these areas and reviewing existing policies.

- **Supporting individuals**

  Union representatives cannot be expected to be qualified counsellors, but often they are the person that you might contact when you have a work-related problem. They can offer support and pointers on where to get help.

How to start a conversation

You may want others to understand what you're going through, but you might feel:

- unable to tell someone
- unsure of who to tell
- concerned that they won't understand
- fearful of being judged
- worried you'll upset them.

If you feel like this, you might not know how to broach the subject with them. One thing you could perhaps do is to show them these pages to help start the conversation and then tell them that you have been thinking about harming yourself.

Suicide helplines

Many countries have suicide helplines and charitable organisations who are:

- Creating a national response to suicide prevention, including a comprehensive multisectoral suicide prevention strategy;
- Restricting access to pesticides, firearms, certain medications and other means of suicide;
- Incorporating suicide prevention as a core component of health-care services; and

Mobilizing communities to provide support to vulnerable individuals, overcome stigma, engage in follow-up care and support those bereaved by suicide.

Whatever you do...

It is important to you ask for help. – you deserve support, you are not alone and there is support out there.

Whether it's a mental health support service, a counsellor or psychotherapist, a union representative, a colleague, a friend, family member or even a pet, telling someone else how you're feeling can help you feel less alone and more in control.

Please share what you are feeling with someone and let them help.

SPACE FOR EXTRA NOTES

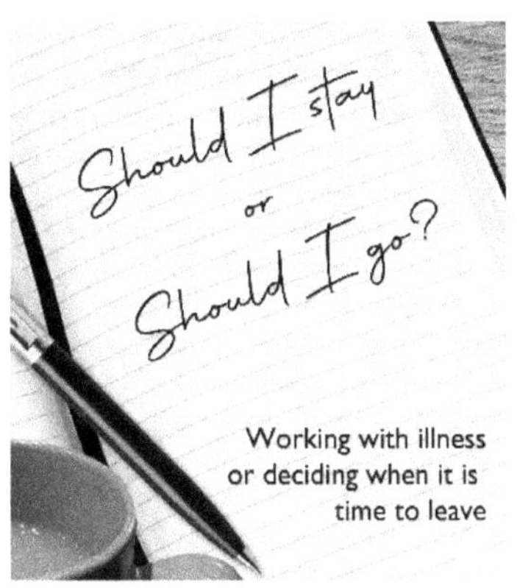

The actual costs of continuing in your role

What are the mental and physical costs of continuing to work rather than staying off work?

- If you have continued to trek into work, how much has this cost you in terms of time, transport and expenses?
- How much has it cost you in terms of your energy and effort – your health levels?
- What has been the mental effect of continuing to work? How are your stress levels?
- Have you felt pressurised to continue working? Who by?

What has been the monetary cost so far of your illness / injury / disability?

- How much have you had to spend during your illness / injury / disability – on seeing doctors, fulfilling prescriptions, medical aids, attending appointments, seeing a specialist, transport to and from (including parking) for all appointments?
- Have you had to have a special diet, or had to have food delivered because you have been unable to shop?
- Have you lost any earnings from being ill?

What has been the time cost of your illness / injury / disability?

- How much time have you taken out from work to attend appointments – including travel to and from?
- How long have you spent waiting for treatments (both in terms of waiting for appointments to become available, and waiting at doctors' clinics)?
- Has your illness / injury / disability caused you to spend longer following your normal daily routine and / or your work?
- How much time has been spent on bed rest, etc?

> **During your time on sick leave, what contact have you had with your company, if any?**

- Have you been plagued by calls for help from your boss or your colleagues?
- Have you been ignored totally?
- Have you been feeling forgotten by your colleagues when off sick, especially if you were the usually the person who arranged flowers and cards for others but no-one has done it for you?
- Are you worrying about what work will face you on your return?
- Are you worried that your time off might affect your role / promotion in the future?

Should you allow / ask work colleagues visit you at hospital or at home or elsewhere while off sick?

- Have colleagues asked to visit you? Or have you asked them?
- On what basis?
- What are the pros and the cons of having a colleague visit you?
- What about the company's ethics, and the moral difficulties which can arise from visits?
- Have you considered gossip which might stem from a visit?

Have you attended any formal or informal meetings relating to your time off?

- Have you been asked to meet with Human Resources personnel or your boss, or anyone else, while you have been off?
- Were you given notice in writing, with the opportunity to bring a representative?
- Have you felt pressured to attend any such meetings?
- Was the purpose of the meeting clearly outlined to you?
- Have there been any consequences since?

Is your company adhering to its sickness procedures and policies?

- Do you know what your statutory rights are, as an employee, relating to taking time off for sick leave or medical treatments?
- And what does your company's procedures and policies offer?
- Are you a member of a Union? If not, can you join now? Ask them for clarity if you are unsure of anything, they are there to assist.

Is your company adhering to its grievance and disciplinary policies?

- Have you got a copy of the policies? If not, get them NOW.
- Is your company taking steps against you because of your time off due to illness / incapacity to carry out your job?
- Ask your Union to help you immediately.
- If you are not already a Union member, join one.
- Is your job threatened by any policies which the company is following?

SPACE FOR EXTRA NOTES

SPACE FOR EXTRA NOTES

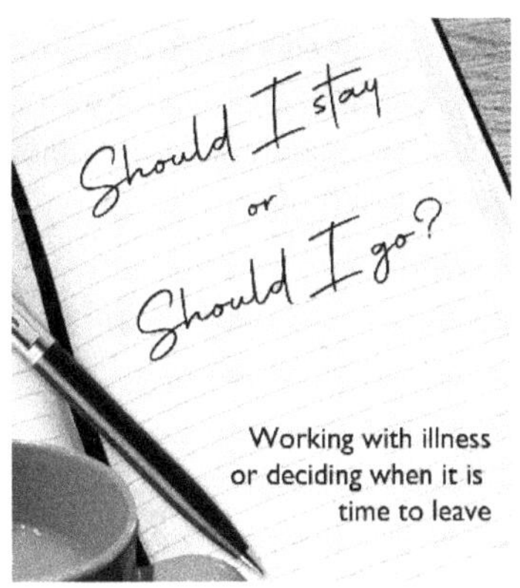

The financial implications of leaving

How is the company managing without you now?

- How is your boss / department / team coping at the moment without you?
- Will they be able to continue to?
- Is there someone ready to step into your role if you leave?
- Have you previously made any 'what to do in your absence' plans at work?
- If you left could you persuade the company to pay you to produce a detailed hand-over folder for your successor?

> **MONEY: What differences are there for you right now, in terms of what you usually earn?**

- How much were you earning before the illness / injury / disability?
- Has this changed, and by how much per week/month?
- What expenses do you have that you need to cover each month – mortgage / rent, food, utility bills, insurance, taxes, etc?
- Are your outgoings more or less since becoming ill / disabled?
- Are you managing financially right now?

MONEY: What would you need, in terms of money, to manage without this job?

- How much do you actually NEED to live on right now?
- Do you need the equivalent of the whole of your salary?
- Could you manage on less, if you were not travelling to work, buying lunches, spending time commuting?
- Do you have health insurance to cover your doctors / medications / treatments?

Notes on leaving your job through ill health – whether resigning, negotiating to leave, taking redundancy, or being dismissed.

Resigning from your job

If you resign, you will be required to work your notice period, although you might be on sick leave during this.

You will automatically lose any benefits of which came with your job, such as:

- Death in service benefit –this will be particularly important when you are seriously ill, even though it may seem a difficult topic
- Pension rights
- Any health insurance or related benefits like gym memberships.

Being ill or becoming disabled is difficult and stressful enough.

It is best to ensure you are not also left in financial difficulty before any decisions are made.

If you stop paying into a private pension or into your country's social security system because you are no longer employed, the amount you have saved to live on when you retire will be less.

Check with a financial advisor before making any decisions that relate to your pension.

Could you negotiate a leaving agreement?

Depending on the level of seniority in your role, if you have been employed for a long time you may be able to negotiate with your employers, which could allow you to keep some of your employment benefits until you are well or able to find alternative work.

Arranging to leave in this way can be mutually beneficial; you get some support short term without the pressure to return, whilst they are free to cover your role.

Get help from your union representative or a lawyer if you going down this route.

Taking redundancy

Discrimination laws in most countries prohibit your employers from making your role redundant because of your illness / disability.

Should your company being asking for voluntary redundancies whilst you are considering leaving work, you may wish to consider this option.

This may be advantageous as you will be paid a final salary and you can negotiate other things you may like to be included in the package.

You will likely be entitled to or better able to negotiate if you have been at a place of work for a long period of time.

Ensure you consider how long any redundancy payment will support you for and make plans for how you will support yourself after this period.

Take advice to ensure you know your rights: Citizens Advice can advise you throughout the redundancy process.

Can your employer dismiss you because of your illness?

There is no straightforward way for a company to let go of an employee due to ill health.

There are five fair reasons to dismiss an employee, they are:

- Misconduct.
- Redundancy.
- Illegality.
- Capability.
- And other substantial reasons.

It's important for the employer to have a procedure in place to avoid claims of discrimination or unfair dismissal.

This may happen if all reasonable adjustments have been considered and the employee is still unable to return to work in the foreseeable future.

Being dismissed

Your employer could initiate dismissal due to medical incapacity, usually after a minimum of 12 months since you became ill.

Dismissal should be a last resort after exhausting other efforts. Employers should remember to consider reasonable adjustments such as flexible working hours, remote working or issuing alternative responsibilities. If they are not able to make reasonable adjustments, then it may be fair to dismiss an ill employee by reason or incapability.

To avoid claims of discrimination, the employer will have to prove that dismissal was fair and as a result of the employee's incapability. This includes evidence of reasonable adjustments made as well as any other opportunities provided to improve the employee's performance or to return them to work.

Before dismissal on grounds of capability due to ill health, the employer should consider the employee's current medical positions, perhaps by contacting their GP (with the employee's permission) for a report on their fitness and any recommendations in relation to working.

Factors which should be considered before dismissal include the:

- Nature of illness.
- Likelihood of reoccurring absences due to ill health.
- Length of absence.
- Length of service.
- Impact on business.
- Impact on other employees.
- Organisation's sickness policy.

The employer should also consider asking an occupational health specialist to carry out a health assessment. Conducting this assessment can confirm what the problem is, how it'll affect the employee's job and when/if they'll be ready to return to work.

BENEFITS: Are you eligible for any benefits from Government?

In some countries, you can claim unemployment benefits if you leave your job due to illness, injury or disability. You would need to provide documentation from your doctor to back up your claim.

What is the case where you are?

- In the UK, if an illness, injury or disability affects looking after yourself or getting around, apply for Personal Independence Payments (PIP) - evaluated on your physical capabilities and mobility issues. PIP is tax free and available to all, in and out of work.
- If you are earning less now, you could apply for Tax Credits.
- If you are not earning, look into applying for Universal Credit.

Have you any other possible sources for income?

- Do you have any savings? This is the "rainy day" you've been putting money away for.
- Could anyone else in your household contribute more towards your expenses?
- Could a relative or friend help out?
- Does your company have a hardship fund?
- Are you a union member? Could they help in any way? Can you join now?
- Would you consider taking out a loan or putting expenses on a credit card to help you get by during your illness?

Are you eligible for any help from elsewhere?

- If you claim benefits, your local council should be able to assist by checking you are receiving all the benefits you could be eligible for.
- Check your Citizen's Advice Bureau website to see if any other help is available to you.
- Some illnesses or disabilities have support associations who may be able to point you towards additional help.

OTHER ASSISTANCE: Can you apply for any additional assistance in kind?

- Could you, for example, apply for assisted transport, a blue badge for parking, a disabled travel card, a mobility vehicle?
- During the Covid19 pandemic in the UK people with certain illnesses or disabilities have been eligible for food parcels and priority delivery slots with supermarkets... Are you eligible any such assistance?
- If you have a pension fund, can you take early retirement on ill health grounds?

SPACE FOR EXTRA NOTES

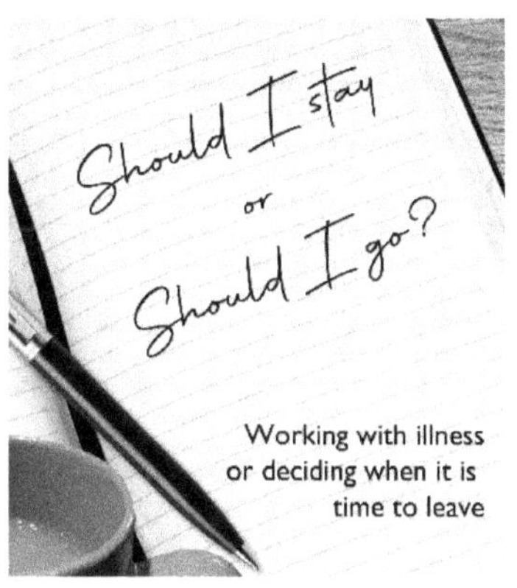

If you leave, what next?

> **What do you want / need to do next if you don't continue in your current job?**

- Current career - could you see yourself working in another role / organisation, in the same industry / career?
- A new career - has your passion for your current industry / career waned - would you prefer a different role entirely?
- Working for yourself – could you develop your own business / work as a freelancer?
- Stopping working - are you a position where you could perhaps retire?

<table>
<tr><td>What skills / training / equipment might you need for the future?</td></tr>
</table>

- Look into what skills or training you might need.
- Would you need any specialised equipment?
- How can you pay for these?
- What possible benefits or schemes might be available to you to pay for training, to keep you in work of some kind, to help make up any shortfall in earnings, to support you?

Some pointers on applying for another job, if you leave your current one through ill health.

- After figuring out what career path you want to pursue, think about the following when writing a new CV and applying for jobs?
- Which skills, abilities and interests from your previous experience can you shift to a new field or job?
- Do you need more training or education for this new perspective, and if so, can you afford to pay for training, especially if you don't work and sustain yourself during the process?
- Are there companies that hire people in this new field that you are trying to enter?
- Are you willing to accept a lower-level position, if necessary?
- Do you have the energy and resistance to manage a potentially stressful job change, after dealing with the physical and emotional trauma that illness can inflict?
- Don't leave a gap on your application / CV, or try to disguise your illness.
- Be sure to highlight any work from home, voluntary work, re-training or freelance work that you have done during your time off.
- Use your covering letter as an opportunity to explain the gap.
- Also use your application covering letter to put forward how this experience has transformed you into a stronger person – for example, able to respond well to a crisis, determination to learn more and upskill yourself during your time off, .better empathy with staff who are suffering problems themselves.

How do you refer in applications or at interview to leaving your last job through ill health?

If you want / need to continue working, how would you refer to leaving your current job when applying / at interview? You need to think about the issue in advance and almost script it out for the interview. You might consider using any or all of the following:

- Give relevant facts about your sick leave that aren't too personal. Give the dates of your time off work, but don't be overly specific with the medical issue.
- 'I had a medical issue and took care of it, and now I'm ready to get back to work.'
- 'I made the very difficult decision to leave my job; now I'm eager to get back to work.'"
- Explain why what you've been through makes you a great employee, how you have dealt with challenges and successfully resolved arising problems.
- Be wary of overpromising what you can deliver given your physical and mental condition.
- Will you need any further time off for additional treatment? Take a list from your doctor or consultant that lists your appointment schedule.
- If you need any specialised equipment / support, give details and demonstrate that you have thought carefully about how you manage a return to work.
- If you have recovered from your condition to an extent that you feel able to work again, you might want to ask your doctor to provide a certificate of fitness of work as evidence.

What else could you be doing instead with your time if you don't continue to work?

- Could this be a well-timed and considered exit, opening a door to new opportunities?
- Do you have any ambitions / hopes / dreams / aspirations which you could maybe look into now?
- Can you afford to maintain your current home and lifestyle?
- Does your pension fund permit early retirement on ill health grounds?
- Do you have savings that could assist or would downsizing provide you with funds?
- Could you downsize your home or move / abroad to be mortgage or rent free?

Some things to consider about attitudes to illness if you are leaving work.

You might want to spend some time thinking through how you will tell people that you are leaving work due to ill health. Be prepared for varied reactions from people who perhaps don't understand your situation.

You could, for example, be worried about people's perceptions about you. Someone might suggest that you haven't thought of all the options, or offer help to find you a job, or "surely there must be something you can do". You might worry that they are judging you or your health condition and coming to incorrect conclusions such as "you look well, surely you must be well enough to go to work of some sort?"

These will, on the most part, be people trying to make helpful suggestions, which may not actually be helpful to you as you will have already exhausted all the options to you. You might have accepted your health condition, but you may find that you also need others to accept it – their "helpful" suggestions can sometimes actually feel hurtful if they do not understand your situation.

There is, of course, the chance that you are imagining what other people are thinking about you, based on your own feelings on your situation.

Making the decision to not actively look for work any more can be the best thing for your health – but please be aware that this could have a big impact on you psychologically, on your self-esteem and emotionally. This is quite common amongst people who need to leave work due to ill health – getting used to our limitations and learning to change our mindset about what we now can and cannot do, can take its toll.

Whatever you decide, you need to be able to accept and come to terms with it – including that you will no longer be a tax-paying working member of society.

You may also have had your own perceptions about ill health in the past – your current condition will be challenging your perceptions now.

Many people can be very dismissive about mental health problems and illness having an impact on someone else in the workplace – often until they suffer from something themselves, and then their perceptions change. Similarly, you may always have felt that you are a very strong character and are able to do anything, but when suddenly faced with incapacity or ill health your vision of your former self can feel compromised and hard to come to terms with.

Accepting your illness / injury / mental health condition / disability is hard enough to do – to then accept that it has such a huge impact on your working life, financial situation, home situation, health and your future can feel even harder at times.

You need to re-evaluate your image of what your future and your retirement were going to be like – you need to change your plans in order to fit your new situation.

This is where you need to ensure that you have a good support mechanism around you – and that you truly believe you have gone through the all of the options thoroughly in coming to your decision.

What has your own attitude been towards illness in the past – and what is it now that you yourself have become ill / disabled?

SPACE FOR EXTRA NOTES

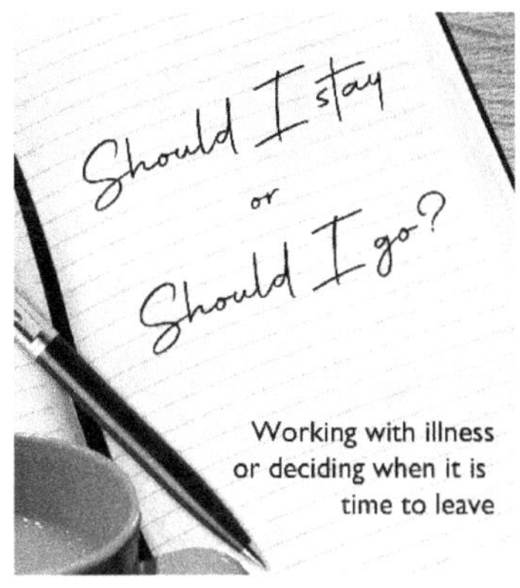

Weighing up your reasons to stay or go

HEALTH AND FINANCES: How important is your health to you, in comparison to your job and your finances - really think about this!

- Could your physical or mental health be affected detrimentally by staying in your job?
- Would you be better off (health-wise) without it?
- Could you manage financially – or could you find a way to manage?
- Which is more important to you – your job / career / finances, or your health?

> **What motivates / urges / pushes / threatens you into feeling you want to or should continue in this job?**

- "I want to stick through it, I want to work hard and win. I want to conquer this disease! I want to make money. I want to fit in and be considered valuable."
- "I need the money / financial security."
- "I love the job and want to continue in it."
- "I'm scared that there is nothing else I can do."
- What would be the benefits to you for staying?
- What effect would this have on your health?

What motivates / urges / pushes / threatens you into feeling you want to or should leave?

- Does this time of being off work give you time to reflect on what you want to do next in life?
- You've had a chance to reassess your priorities.
- This is an opportunity for you to follow a lifelong dream or ambition, or just time for a welcome change.
- This gives you an opening to step down from a higher level role to something less taxing and stressful.

Some final thinking points on leaving your job.

- Deciding to stay or go is a big decision that effects not only your current finances but also those in the future, for you and your family. Therefore, it is advisable to take financial and legal advice alongside the advice of your doctor before you make the decision and give yourself enough time to do so after diagnosis.
- Taking action to help ourselves is crucial, but it's also incumbent on society to provide a method to accommodate this; on employers to truly be humane and flexible; and on each one of us to catch ourselves when we judge another.
- We should feel empowered to make these choices. We should feel inspired and strengthened by making a difficult decision. And we should work against those sending those messages around value and worth.
- Leaving your job doesn't necessarily mean that you can't work, or won't be able to work ever again. It might simply mean that you need to find what works best for you right now.
- Leaving your job can bring a sense of loss. You may need to spend time grieving the fact that you couldn't focus on being your best at work and had to instead focus on getting better.
- On the other hand, leaving your job can bring a sense of joy. For the first time in a long time, you could be on your route toward healing in the light of new productivity and happiness, and learning what your personal limits and necessities really are.

Where can you find out more information on any issue brought up within this book?

You could consider contacting:

- your doctor's surgery
- your hospital or any clinics that you have attended
- your local Adult Social Care team
- your local benefits office
- your local employment service
- the local Citizen's Advice Bureau.

You should talk with:

- your immediate family – how will your decision impact upon your home, your partnership, your children?
- Friends, family or contacts who have been through similar situations
- your boss (if they are amenable!)
- your Human Resource department
- your Union representative
- your employment service contact
- trusted colleagues
- the administrators of your pension fund
- a financial advisor
- a counsellor or psychotherapist.

Look further on the internet for:

- reputable medical sources of information about your condition
- Facebook groups on your illness / injury / disability
- associations / support groups / helplines for your condition
- your local labour laws and conditions.
- All of these could contribute towards your decision-making.

USE THESE PAGES TO ASSIST WITH YOUR DECISION MAKING

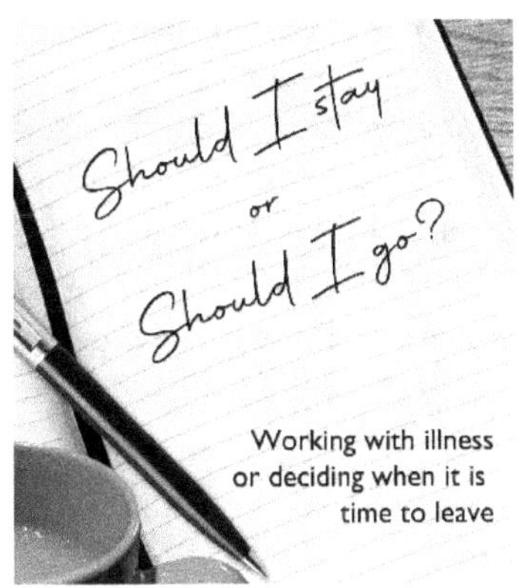

Case studies: personal decisions

About the case studies:

Hopefully on reaching this point in the book you are now feeling more secure about your own decision-making process regarding your future.

This section shares the decision-making processes (and outcomes, where possible) of around twenty individuals who have all experienced some form of illness, injury, mental health problem or disability, and have had to come to some sort of decision about their future employment possibilities. Some have continued in their jobs, others have moved to alternative roles or changed career entirely, some have set up their own business, some have retired from working and some have even moved country. They have all agreed to share their stories.

These case studies come from several sources:

- my own experience
- my friends, family, colleagues and contacts
- individuals who have written internet blogs about their experiences, and
- the UK's 'Employment Advisors in Improving Access to Psychological Therapy' (EAs in IAPT) contract.

Many of the case studies have been written by the individuals themselves, others have been written by myself or the IAPT service on their behalf.

A note on Data Protection and Anonymisation:

Permission to include these stories has been sought – and received from - each person. Several have given permission to use their full names and details in their stories, whilst others have asked for anonymity so I have changed names, locations and other details as required.

The IAPT case studies were provided to me having already been anonymised by the service, and with consent having been gathered from the individuals involved.

Each of the blog posts include their author's web address, and contain their real names.

ANGELA GARRY

Leaving full-time work to concentrate on a part-time business from home

"Writing this book has come about as a result of my own decision-making process a few years ago.

"I was working in a full-time job, with 10 to 12 hour days, sitting at a desk working on a computer. In free time and vacations I developed and delivered training courses for administrative staff worldwide.

"Due to an illness which I had been managing for a couple of years I had a surgery which unfortunately left me with severe back pain. High-strength painkillers left me feeling dizzy, nauseous and extremely tired, plus they didn't alleviate the back pain so much as just make me not care about it – and they made it impossible for me to drive to work. I was unable to concentrate on anything for more than half an hour, let alone 10 to 12 hours a day, so I couldn't have continued to do my job. Without the painkillers though I could not sit at either a desk to do my job or in my car (or any other mode of transport) for the 10 mile journey to work.

"My doctor signed me off work for several months and the longer that time went on I realised I would not be able to return to my job as my back pain was not getting better. For a while I tried to ignore this as I loved my job and wanted to return to it – but eventually I started to think about what I could do if I left. The questions that I asked myself became part of this book.

"I knew I could bring in some money from bits of part-time work from my home – creating one-off training programmes, selling distance learning courses and writing/editing articles for a magazine – plus I wanted to write a book.

"My back pain and subsequent walking problems became legally considered a 'disability' in the UK after several months, making me eligible to receive Personal Independence Payments (PIP), a benefit for those suffering from a disability. This added a small element of financial security for me and I worked out that if I was careful with money I should be able to manage if I left my job to work for myself part-time from home, particularly as the spare time I would then have would allow me to market my training programmes more.

"I left my full-time job because of my back pain in early 2014. Since then I have had more physiotherapy plus chiropractic treatment, along with Reiki and EFT ('tapping') and I've weaned myself off the high-strength painkillers. I now use a range of other methods to help manage the back pain so that I can sit for longer periods. During the last seven years I have worked part-time for myself as an author / editor (dictating almost 30 books into my phone or laptop). I'm also a practicing psychotherapist, and continue to develop and deliver training for administrative staff.

"A separate serious illness in 2016 reduced my breathing capacity and energy levels – and in 2020 I sold my house to move to Spain where the warmer climate is much better for my health, including my back pain and arthritis. The move has been a continuation of my process, doing whatever I can to work with my disability."

TERRI-ANNE DYLAN

Moving from full-time in a school to part-time in a number of schools

Terri-Anne was a teacher in a secondary school where she felt bullied by several of the colleagues in her department, including the Department Head.

When timetabling was created at the beginning of each school year, Terri-Anne believed she was deliberately given the worst classes, whilst the Department Head and their favourite teachers were timetabled to work with the easier groups of pupils.

In Department meetings she felt that her point of view was deemed irrelevant and she was not given space to bring topics for discussion, plus her input in other discussions was ignored or were undermined. Her efforts in several extra-curricular activities went un-recognised, and she felt that there was an attempt to push her out of the Department entirely.

She spoke with the Department Head who vehemently denied everything, even though Terri-Anne had made thorough notes of incidents and instances where she had felt bullied and pressurised within the department.

After four and a half years, the stress and strain caused Terri-Anne to see her doctor when she had woken one morning to find that the mere thought of going to work in the school filled her with dread and made her feel physically ill. She was tearful and felt nauseous the whole time. The doctor immediately signed her off from work for several weeks on grounds of workplace stress.

The weeks off turned into months, and Terri-Anne sought help from a therapist to talk through her mental health problems. She fully realised that these stemmed directly from the stress she was under at work.

During the months away from the school, Terri-Anne started to feel much better in herself – but every time she thought of returning to work she became ill again.

She came to realise that she needed to leave the school in order to regain her mental health.

Instead of taking on a new role full-time in another school she weighed up the monetary costs of working full-time against her own physical and mental needs - and joined a teaching supply agency, working a few days per week in various schools as and when she was needed.

These other schools and their departments have all reacted really positively to Terri-Anne and have loved both her and her work. This has given her the feeling of stability that she had craved – the feeling of being needed, of being useful, of being appreciated in her work.

NOELEEN ALDRIDGE

Working shift patterns caused her to move country

"I worked for Intel in Ireland in a fabrication plant making microchips.

For the first three years I worked 7 pm to 7. 20 am and then my shifts changed to one month on days then one month on nights.

Other than during food breaks, I wore full body protection similar to what you see astronauts wearing. This dehydrates you and makes you feel very tired.

Initially I loved working nights but eventually I lost the ability to sleep as I was concentrating at work on trying to stay awake when my body thought I should be sleeping and vice versa.

Needless to say, I hit a wall and eventually left the job to move to Spain almost 16 years ago.

I have tried varying tactics to get my sleep pattern back but have never fully succeeded.

Life throws curveballs but I prefer to be here to keep on a straight line."

JULIETTA DANCY

Making changes in the workplace and shortening her working hours

"Before all this happened, I worked in an insurance company on the third floor of a four-storey building without a lift, in the middle of the city. Parking my car anywhere nearby was always a nightmare and I used to end up parking way out of town and getting the' Park and Ride' bus which then left me with a ten to fifteen minute walk to the office. In wet weather I loathed it.

Then ten years ago I had a car accident one morning where a truck driver didn't see my car and pulled out into my car. The truck smashed into the driver's side of my car and I had to be cut from the wreckage.

I was really lucky to survive the impact, but my right leg was badly damaged and I've had three surgeries on it since. I was off work for several months. This was before the days when many companies allowed staff to work from home – and I was bored rigid at home whilst I was recuperating between the surgeries!

Returning to work was an interesting experience – I had to have a few phone calls with my boss to see how we could manage things. One of the first things to look as was how I could get to work and then if I could get to the building how would I get to my office, because there was no lift and I couldn't get to the toilets on the next floor.

Eventually we worked it out how I could get to the building – I got a mobility car that I can drive without needing to use my damaged leg and my boss asked the local council to paint a Disabled parking bay on the road specifically for me. I have a lightweight folding wheelchair which I can manage, so that all meant I could physically get to work. There was already a ramp at the front door, so that meant I could get inside. But what about my office?

I worked as part of a small team, and the boss organised for two teams to switch places in the building – one team moved up to the third floor and my team moved down to their previous space on the ground floor, just down the corridor from the disabled toilet. This made it easy for me to get to my job and work on the ground floor, whilst able to remain independent in doing so.

So now we're ten years on and I'm still working in the job that I love. Most days I still need to use the wheelchair to get about, and my energy levels are much reduced, so I work shorter hours now to fit in with my needs. There are some days when I can walk slowly – but not very far, but that's OK, I manage very well with the wheelchair. I'm on my third one now, I wore the other out!

I've realised that this is how things will remain for me. Mentally, I've come to terms with it and I just get up and carry on with things because this is my life now, there's no changing it.

Before the accident getting to work was a chore. At least now I can get to work much easier, because I have a mobility car and my own parking space right outside the building I have a much shorter commute – no driving to the "Park and Ride" then getting a bus and walking in the rain. And because of the shorter hours and the shorter commute, I get more time to spend with my husband who retired two years ago!

There's always a silver lining, I say…"

BRENDAN WILSON

Leaving the Armed Forces due to PTSD

Brendan served in the Armed Forces for several years, including two tours in Afghanistan. He was put on medical sick leave after an incident which left him with Post Traumatic Stress Disorder (PTSD).

After several months on leave, Brendan was offered a rehabilitation programme but found that attending it made him worse because it was aimed at preparing him to return to the Armed Forces, something which filled him with fear.

Eventually Brendan accepted an early pension from the Army, on ill health grounds. At this point Brendan was 38, and his wife Lily 33.

Lily was pregnant when they moved home to a new area, hoping to make a new start. After the birth of their son, Brendan's PTSD became worse – he was incredibly over-protective and didn't want the family to go outside.

He was terrified by news reports from around the world of troubles which prompted thoughts of having to return to active service, something that he couldn't face.

Brendan was on hyper-alert at all times – just the sound of a car door slamming in the street outside his home would make his heart race as if he was engaging in battle.

He found it almost impossible to sleep, and spent hours watching over their baby son, panicking that the child would stop breathing at any moment.

His relationships with Lily and their child suffered. When their child was six years old Lily started to become withdrawn, nervous and anxious.

She had been caring for Brendan since he left the Armed Forces, as well as looking after their child, and the stress became too much for her. She started to worry whether that her constant tiredness and irritability were symptoms of cancer and several other diseases, but all medical tests came back negative.

When Lily approached their doctor for sleeping pills for herself and was referred for short-term therapy to overcome her anxiety, Brendan recognised that he needed to do something about his own mental health and approached the doctor for help.

Brendan was referred to a PTSD clinic where he attends therapy on a weekly basis. For some time he felt unable to apply for any sort of job – but he feels that his life with his wife and child is much more on track again. This came about when he realised that he had been worrying for several years that he might at some point have to return to active service. He now recognised that this is no longer the case, and has been able to see a better future ahead.

In 2020 some of his fears about his family's safety returned during the Covid-19 pandemic, but he has been able to acknowledge these and talk about them with his therapist, who he has been working with via video link.

Brendan has been renovating the family home during the pandemic and says he is now looking forward to finding some form of paid manual work such as carpentry or gardening where he would feel useful but will not constantly be under stress.

EMMA TAYLOR

Leaving work and finding faith

"When I was living in the UK I had been working for a well-known insurance company for years but I suffered with depression and panic attacks.

As they got worse I found I was needing to take more days off sick. I was put on a high dose of medication and saw counsellors to try and help me.

I had to face a lot of stigma about it all, and also had to deal with people not understanding me.

One friend said I needed to leave as I was on my last warning and they felt that working for the company wasn't helping my health.

After more than 7 years I left and a new-found friend introduced to me the church.

My faith pulled me through and I started doing lots of charity work including for my church and a place called 4YP that helps people from 12 to 25 with homelessness and various different things.

I stayed in the UK for a bit before deciding to come out to Spain to start a new life.

Within weeks of being in Spain I was completely anti-depressant free.

I still suffer with anxiety and panic attacks, but luckily the attacks are rare and I now try and speak to people when I'm down."

DAVE PROCTOR

Retiring to Spain after cancer treatments

"I worked with my wife Karen in England, where we had a sports photography business. We had been running this quite successfully for about 10 years and had many repeat customers and were well thought of.

"Then in 2014, I started getting some unusual symptoms regarding my 'movements'. I went to the doctor and he diagnosed piles.

"The symptoms continued and even got worse and like most blokes, I simply ignored these problems and carried on.

"It was after work one evening and 'Doc Martin' starring Martin Clunes was on TV in the background when I hear the main character say to one of his patients 'No-one died of a diagnosis'. This struck home and I returned to my Doctor, who then referred me for a biopsy and cancer was found.

"For the next few months of 2015, I went through the mill of Radiotherapy, chemotherapy and finally a six-hour operation.

"I had a couple of weeks in the hospital and then after a short period of recuperation, I returned to work well before I should have.

"The operation left me substantially weaker and unable to lift (the way we operated was we had printers etc which we took with us).

"We both agreed that we could not continue and weighed up the options and decided that using some creative accounting, we could afford to retire to Spain. We ended up buying a house in a lovely village on the east coast.

"After having all these treatments, needless to say many of which were life-altering and some of which never seemed to get better, I went into depression.

"Apart from my happy pills, as a self-prescription, I then started writing comedy to cheer myself up and surprisingly people thought it was really good.

"My first book, I initially self-published but is now coming out with a London publisher and I have another novel ready to go.

"To also fill my time, I started writing for theatre and within a few weeks had signed with an agency.

"Financially the Covid19 pandemic has meant there has been little income from writing (apart from when I worked as a reporter for a weekly newspaper), but sometimes money is not what it is all about.

"Oh, and I woke up this morning, which was great!"

SLOANE

Leaving her first job due to stress

(reproduced with permission from an article by Anna Marie Houlis at *https://fairygodboss.com/articles/5-ways-to-tell-if-your-job-is-making-you-sick-literally*)

Sloane was just out of business school when she took her first job as a marketing director for what she thought was an "awesome" boutique cosmetics brand, but she later discovered that the company was completely dysfunctional, she says.

The core tenets and leadership style native to her workplace were adversely affecting her health — the stress of it all had even manifested physically.

"There was insane infighting among the management, and the women in charge were downright mean," she explains.

"I made the mistake of speaking up about it to HR and they forced me out of my job and left me to find another position somewhere else within the organization."

Sloane says she was always a star performer at work so she couldn't believe that, in essence, she'd been fired. It was ultimately one of the most stressful experiences of her life, and it was one that took a toll on her skin.

"Suddenly, I broke out in miserably, itchy hives all over my body," she remembers.

"I was covered in them, and they wouldn't go away. They lasted nine weeks. I tried everything: antibiotics, seven doctors and tons of steroids that gave me moon face."

Finally, she'd tried acupuncture and Chinese herbs; the hives started to go away the very next day, but it was a long, enduring journey.

Sloane eventually landed a new job with "some of the best people" she's ever worked with, but not before she'd learned that poor leadership, catty co-workers and an overall corrupt office culture could make one sick — literally. And hives, like Sloane's, aren't the only side affect of negative vibes at work.

"The main reason we might actually start to feel physically ill by being [stuck in bad jobs] is that the amount of stress they put us through ends up manifesting itself in the form of illness or ailments — and the reason why we start to feel ill after being exposed to stress for too long is because our body releases specific hormones to help us deal with stress when we encounter it," explains Caleb Backe, a health and wellness expert for Maple Holistics.

"When we stress, our body releases a mixture of cortisol, epinephrine and norepinephrine to help increase our heart rate and allow us to deal with the stressful events as they occur (i.e. fight or flight mode). While this 'survival mode' has allowed us to survive for thousands of years as a species, it's not something we would want to have to experience every single day."

Backe urges employees not to normalize things that are unacceptable — that's considered "Stockholm Syndrome," he says, and it's something we should all avoid at all costs, especially at our places of work. Of course, that's easier said than done.

NIKKI ALBERT

On finding fulfilment after giving up her career due to fibromyalgia

(reproduced with permission from *https://brainlessblogger.net/2018/01/16/making-life-shine-without-work*)

3 Ways I'm Finding Fulfilment After My Illness Made Me Leave My Career

Chronic illness doesn't eradicate ambition, desires, goals and dreams. But it can limit our capacity to achieve ambitions we have geared our lives for. Careers we aimed for, trained for, had, wanted, lived for… just limited. To the point we can only work casually, part-time or not at all. But it doesn't stop us from having ambitious thoughts.

From seeing those mountains that we cannot climb. And it can be immensely frustrating to know we cannot achieve certain goals. Cannot have certain dreams. Are not permitted certain ambitions?

Giving up a certain career can be a massive blow to our self-worth. Who are we without what we do? How do we have fulfilment in our lives without the career that held some sort of meaning for us? Kept us engaged and interested? Held our goals and ambitions? Our purpose? Our future aims and desires? Our financial stability? How do we find fulfilment with that void there?

Chasing gleams of sunshine, my friends, chasing sunshine.

I do not hold all the answers to this with my damaged self-worth and difficult time coping with this vary issue. Seeing mountains everywhere I want to climb and very aware I cannot. Trying to convince myself I can, and just falling down.

It hurts, that fall, it really, really hurts. But I know a few things.

I chase gleams of sunshine through the following:

1. Keep myself interested and engaged. So I lost a career that was interesting and engaging. This is important. I lack this now. I need something to replace it. We all need something

to keep us interested. So we have to fill that void. I fill it with this blog and my creative writing. So a hobby. Something I have a passion for I can throw myself into. Something I find interesting and engaging.

2. I chase smaller dreams. I make smaller goals and chase smaller ambitions. I try to anyway. I want to have ambitions. I want to have goals and dreams. I just have to make them reasonable and achievable. Focus on what I am capable of instead of what I am clearly not capable of. I want to create something from what I am capable of. Find some sort of niche there.

3. I realized life is about more than work. Work is a small fraction of what life is about and what it should be about. And if everyone knew this, they would be better off. We just need to focus on the aspects of life that are meaningful beyond the job we have or don't have. Our friends, spouse, children and families. Our connections. Our interests. Focus on the meaningful things we do have in our life.

By no means is any of that easy. I want to stretch my limits, knowing the consequences. What happened to my health recently with this massive vestibular flare is a rather epically large print message to my mind that I have health issues aside from pain. That I have limits. That I cannot exceed them because I won't get far and I will regret it, like I always do.

Desire and want don't equal physically capable. No matter how much I wish, desire, want, no matter that I'm mentally and intellectually capable, or that I'm willing. They just don't equal physical capability.

A part of me hates that and therefore doesn't find satisfaction in what I am capable of. Belittles what I am capable of. Mocks it. Says I am worth less because of it. Which is something I, and none of us, should do.

There is value in all the things we are capable of doing. We just need to see the worth in what we do, and the value in our lives as they are now. And find the fulfilment there is to be found in there.

Chase those gleams of sunshine and make them shine, my friends. Make them shine.

KERRY HECKMAN

Taking a part-time role was never in her career plan

(reproduced with permission from
https://globallymealliance.org/grieving-loss-career-chronic-illness)

For an educator, the start of the school year is filled with energy and excitement. There are students to meet, classrooms to decorate, and co-workers to catch up with. There is an undefinable sense of hope that comes with a new beginning.

This fall, for the first time in ten years, when all the other educators went back to work, I wasn't with them. Instead, I was at sitting at home watching the steady stream of "first day of school" pictures on my computer. My career as a school social worker was cut short by Lyme disease.

Two years ago, I thought I would have my job until I retired. It's rare for someone to give up tenure, a pension, affordable health insurance, paid sick days, and summers off. However, this year I opted for a part-time job as a college counsellor to focus on healing. I never thought I would be the person who checks the "part-time" box on questionnaires. My entire identity was wrapped up in my career.

I know I'm not alone. I've heard countless stories of teachers, doctors, and successful business people who were forced to leave behind a thriving career when illness struck. The careers they had worked their entire lives to build were suddenly gone or placed on permanent hold. Last year the mayor of Monticello, Illinois, resigned due to complications of Lyme disease. When he resigned at a town council meeting, he said, "I do this with great regret. It's one of the hardest things I've had to do."

I couldn't agree more.

Leaving my job was truly the hardest decision I've ever made. This past summer, I agonized over whether or not to go back. I loved my job and I was making enough money so that I wouldn't have to worry about the high cost of Lyme treatment. I'd developed lifelong friendships with co-workers and every day I got to make a difference in the lives of young people. On the other hand, I wasn't getting any better, in fact I was getting worse. On a typical weekday I went from my bed, to work, to the couch, back to bed. I was living half a life.

I'd known other people who left jobs due to illness, and I always thought, "That will never be me. I will never get to that point." I worked through the worst two years of my illness. The first year I missed 14 days of school because of doctor's appointments, being bedridden and a hospitalization. The second year I pushed through the year only to crash for an entire month of the summer. For the last two years, the beginning of the school year felt less like returning home and more like a shift back into stress, fatigue and pain.

For people with chronic Lyme disease there comes a point where you can't do the things you used to do. You may not be able to work, engage in creative pursuits, or even socialize anymore. For some people the reality is disability and incapacitation. The difficulty is compounded because Lyme is an invisible illness and outsiders don't understand why you can't work. Other people think not working or working less is a gift. They don't think about the terrible suffering, the symptoms of the illness, or the fact that many people actually want to work. They want to make a contribution to their family's financial and emotional security and feel like they have a purpose in life.

When there is a loss, you need to go through a grieving process. You need to allow yourself to be sad, confused, and even angry. For me, it's difficult, because I don't know what to call myself anymore. I hold a social work license, but I'm not doing social work. I have to grieve the loss of what could have been, then find a way to move beyond it.

Recently, I've started walking a labyrinth in a nature preserve by my house. It's a walking meditation where you walk along a circular path. It has many switchbacks and turn arounds, but you're always moving closer to the centre. I'd heard of labyrinths as a place to go when you're going through a difficult time in your life. The first time I walked the labyrinth was shortly after I left my job. As I was walking the path one day, I realized it was a metaphor for life. There are setbacks and times you need to turn around and retrace your steps, but even so, you are always making progress. I didn't know what was at the end of the labyrinth; when I got to the centre, the word "hope" was spelled out in a mosaic. No matter where your life takes you, no matter the losses you must endure, whether it be illness, the loss of a job, or the loss the life you thought you'd have, it's important to know at the centre of it all is that tiny word, hope.

Hope like the first day of school.

The final stage of the grieving process is often referred to as "acceptance and hope." During this stage we stop wishing for the life we used to have and accept the new normal. Maybe one day I will go back to being a full-time social worker, or maybe not. Right now, I'm trying to look at the loss of my career, not as a loss, but as a beginning. Maybe my job needed to go away in order for me to find a different path, a better path.

Chronic illness has changed me. It changed the way I see the world and changed my goals. Even if the only goal right now is just to get better, I can't think of a more noble one than that.

The following case studies have been submitted by Ally Campbell, Team Manager for EA in IAPT at Ingeus in Derbyshire, England.

She has sought and received consent from seven clients of the service to share their decision-making stories. They have all had particularly interesting journeys regarding decisions to stay, leave, or change work.

Their stories have been written by Ally from a service perspective, using notes from the clients' appointments plus input from their employment advisors.

EA in IAPT Case study 1

Not in employment (exited with outcome in a new industry)

This client had been made redundant following a restructure and had anxiety and trust issues with employers following this and previous experiences.

She had worked in a commercial environment for years, but prior to that had enjoyed public sector work.

She felt her skillset and experience meant she should apply for similar commercial jobs, however repeatedly expressed that she was compromising herself in these roles – that whilst she was good at them and they paid well, she wanted a greater purpose than to just make money for a big company, and she was often treated her poorly and kept being unhappy.

She was referred to our service whilst receiving IAPT therapy for anxiety and depression and wanted to be working again.

She knew the financial and mental health benefits of working but also wanted to protect herself from another bad experience, and was scared that the wrong employer would impact her mental health further now or cause a relapse in the future.

Her employment advisor explored her work related anxieties, and gave her tools and techniques to keep herself well in work, developed her confidence boundary setting with managers, and helped her understand her skillset and value in the context of other job types and industries.

Together they discussed possible jobs that would give her a greater sense of purpose and reward, and also discussed financial requirements and other considerations.

She applied for a number of jobs and secured a management role in a public service – using a lot of her skills and experience from her commercial roles in a way that has a positive impact on other people, which aligns much more closely with her values.

Making the decision to leave an industry she knew and start something unknown was difficult and scary, however she also knew that choosing to stay in it and start another new role that didn't make her happy would not help her depression and anxiety either.

Her employment advisor and therapist helped her work through the factors that were holding her back, and gave her the confidence and support to make a big but beneficial change.

> ## EA in IAPT Case study 2
> ## Employed and in work (on programme)

This client was employed and working when referred to the service, however had already decided she wanted to find new work and had been trying alone without success.

The client was early in her IAPT therapy though had made some initial realisations and was working to regain control, as she considered multiple changes regarding her home life and the future of her marriage as well as her career.

The client has been in her current role for two years but feels unchallenged by the role, has uncertainty about the future of the business, and sees no career progression for herself with this company.

The client had applied for and interviewed for a few roles before joining the EA in IAPT service, however kept just missing out on getting the role. This was frustrating but the client was focused on her goal of securing new work, as she knew her current position was no longer suitable for her.

Her employment advisor discussed potential progression opportunities within the company that the client had not thought of, and supported her to have the discussion with her employer.

The employment advisor also supported her to edit her CV, both focus and widen her job search, and engage with learning opportunities offered by her union.

Whilst in our service the client's line manager left a new one started which was actually positive for the client, however she remained focused on the longer term benefits of securing a new job – career progression, a more certain company future, and a new and more challenging role.

She has attended more interviews though has been unsuccessful in securing new work, and her employment advisor continues to support her with job search, interview skills relating to feedback she receives, and building resilience and maintaining motivation through setbacks.

EA in IAPT Case study 3

Employed and in work (on programme)

This client has been working for his current company for 9 years, and was promoted into a leadership role.

He recently stepped down from this position as he found the career progression and salary increase was not worth the extra stress he experienced, and his employer supported this move for his wellbeing.

He says he's known for a while that he needs to make a job change for his wellbeing and financial concerns, but has been putting it off.

Following an accident the client has a lower limb amputation and uses a prosthesis which can cause discomfort, though he is not physically limited in his ability to do most jobs.

At referral to our service he feels his IAPT treatment has not yet been beneficial and he is changing to a different therapist and therapy type.

His employment advisor explored his work experience prior to this company and helped him recognise his varied skillset, as well as discussing what types of work the client enjoys.

Together they explored various roles and industries, and discussed how some of the jobs he is skilled and experienced for do not meet his financial requirements or require him to work hours that conflict with his family responsibilities.

They also discussed potential training that may open more opportunities for the client to progress his career without taking on leadership duties.

The employment advisor and client are both job searching and reviewing the suitability of a range of roles against what the client wants as well as how well he meets the application criteria.

The employment advisor has supported the client to write a CV that showcases his transferable skills and will run mock interviews with the client to prepare him for any interviews he secures.

Currently the job market in his industry is mainly temporary and seasonal vacancies, which is not an appropriate move him for him.

Whilst the client has financial and wellbeing motivations to change job he feels stable in his current role until he find the right permanent role for him, and his employment advisor will support him both towards securing the new job and staying well in his current job until then.

-155-

EA in IAPT Case study 4

Employed and in work (on programme)

This client had been with her employer for 5 years when she was referred to our service by her therapist, and enjoyed the job and responsibilities.

After disclosing and requesting support relating to her mental health, her manager began to micromanage her work, gave conflicting priorities, and communicated with her either through formal processes or by rearranging her diary without notice or explanation.

 The client was confused, frustrated, and concerned by the manager's intentions, explaining this pattern had happened before to a colleague in a similar position who ended up leaving the organisation.

The client felt like she had little control over her own workload or the way her employer was responding to her mental health disclosure, which was all impacting her mental health further.

The employment advisor supported the client to raise concerns about how the employer was managing her work and mental health disclosure, and suggested reasonable adjustments to her manager's approach that would benefit both the client's mental health and productivity in work.

This achieved some clarifications however the client distrusted management and lacked motivation to rebuild relationships and workload in her current job.

She realised she had achieved all she could within this role and did not see any career progression for herself at that company.

The client began job searching for roles that were more interesting or required her to develop her skills, to make a positive step forward in her career, and also told her employer she was open to a role change within the company if anything suitable came up.

The client continued to receive conflicting priorities, unclear instructions, and tasks with deadlines too short to meet, and her mental health declined.

 After discussing finances and her mental health with her partner and employment advisor the client resigned from her job, intending to rest and focus on her mental health recovery whilst seeking new work.

The employment advisor continues to support to the client in searching for relevant temporary and suitable permanent roles, tailoring her CV and writing cover letters for applications, and in building resilience and maintaining motivation for her next career step.

EA in IAPT Case study 5

Employed and in work (on programme)

This client was approaching his 20 year anniversary at work, which was celebrated with a paid bonus, however was wanting to leave the job due to a new manager and a conflicting working style.

The client felt undermined and overly criticised by his new manager, who contacts him outside of his working hours, and found out he wasn't the only one.

He was referred into our service by his therapist, and wanted support to achieve his 20 year bonus and then leave the job in a planned way and on positive terms, potentially to go part time or take early retirement.

The employment advisor supported the client to prepare for and have conversations with HR and his manager, and signposted him to further support services (CAB, ACAS, and a local law centre should it be required in future).

As these conversations progressed the client had an opportunity to write a proposal for a restructure for his department, in response to other staff leaving and a need to modernise.

He included a change in the requirements for his role and therefore the chance for him to take voluntary redundancy.

His employment advisor researched and provided information on voluntary redundancy for him to consider and discuss the reality of this option before submitting the proposal, and discussed what career options he had open to him if her were to leave the company sooner than expected.

The restructure proposal was approved and the client achieved paid gardening leave as well as their 20 year bonus within their voluntary redundancy agreement.

The client is now developing owned property for holiday rental, volunteering in an area of interest, and looking into part time work options in this field.

His employment advisor will support him through the transitional period of leaving work and with applying for suitable positions.

EA in IAPT Case study 6

Employed and off work (exited with outcome)

This client was referred to our service by her therapist after a new manager became very controlling of her work and forced changes in her working hours, and regularly contacted our client outside of work hours.

The client was anxious and wanted support looking for new work, and was signed off work by her GP for anxiety and depression. She did not want to be signed off work, though her employment advisor helped her see how this time off could be used to her benefit.

Whilst signed off her employment advisor discussed her current role and manager, the pros and the cons of staying and leaving, and what reasonable adjustments could be requested if she were to try to stay.

The client proposed a different shift pattern to her manger which she felt would be more manageable in terms of both her workload and her mental health.

This was accepted, and the employment advisor supported her in her return to work and with techniques to stay well in work.

The client had also expressed interest in self employment which the employment advisor supported her to explore further, and the client enrolled in online training to refresh her skills in that area and agreed a workspace with her landlord.

This client had complex support needs in her therapy, including domestic abuse and housing issues.

Whilst working with her employment advisor this escalated and the client was hospitalised and the police became involved.

After returning to her part time job, starting her online course, and planning her own business start-up, the client expressed gratitude to her employment advisor for their support.

She stated that thanks to him she now feels positive, feeling in control of her own destiny and equipped to deal with decisions and circumstances that are out of her control.

EA in IAPT Case study 7

Employed and in work (exited with outcome)

This client was employed when referred by her therapist, however was in the middle of a complex situation at work.

She had reported a colleague for serious misconduct at work who was dismissed as a result and then reinstated following an appeal.

The client and another colleague were the target of in work bullying by this individual on their return, which was not well managed by the employer.

The client wanted help securing a new role so she could leave this one, and support in her current role until she was able to leave.

Once job searching the client identified there were limited opportunities for her job role in her area, and her employment advisor approached the idea of staying in her current role.

After discussion the client decided she did not want to feel forced out of a job that was otherwise great for her, and her employment advisor focused support on resolving the in work issues and supporting the client to lead this.

Her employment advisor also signposted her to ACAS and a local law centre to access further information on employment rights and grievances.

Alongside this the client's work was impacted by covid19 regulations, as her employer required her to wear a mask in work despite being medically exempt due to the mask triggering her PTSD.

The client proposed a visor alternative however her manger refused, and the employment advisor signposted her to the local law centre who advised on covid19 related employee rights.

Her employment advisor extended in work support to included coping strategies for anxiety relating to wearing the mask and helped the client prepare for mask conversations, which led to her employer completing risk assessments and approving the use of a visor instead of a mask.

The client reached a suitable position in work regarding her relationship with her manager and no contact with the problematic colleague, and was happy she had been able to stay in her job.

During her employment support she had also explored longer term career plans, including her employment advisor identifying skills she already had that would support her ideas and building her confidence in her ability to achieve them, and sourcing information on training for her to take the next steps.

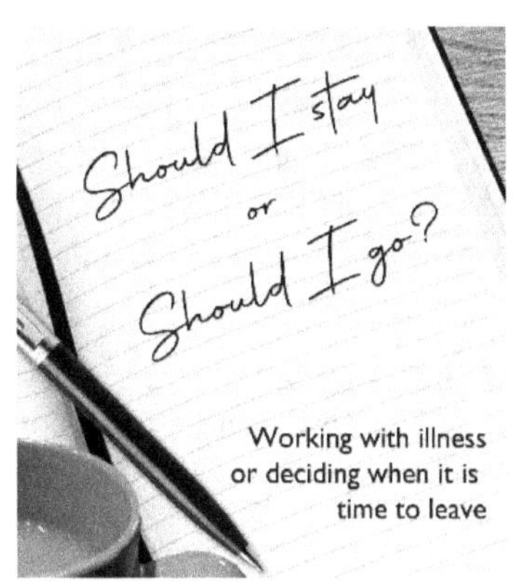

Your decision

Your decision

Only you will know, from how you have felt and what you have thought about during the completion of this book, whether you WANT to stay in your job or would PREFER to go.

Hopefully going through each and every section will have assisted you in making the actual DECISION as to what's best for you and your family – and possibly also for your company and your boss.

In the next section are a number of case studies from individuals – true stories of people making their own decisions about whether they can (or should) stay in their role or find another path.

So – what have you decided?   Are you going to

STAY or GO?

Good luck, either way!

Angela Garry

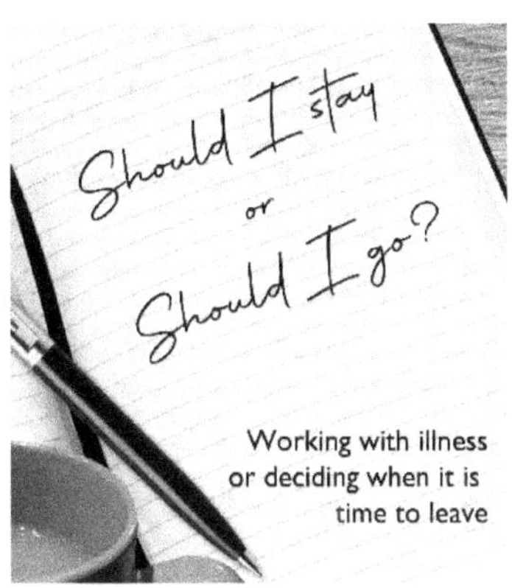

About the Author

About the Author

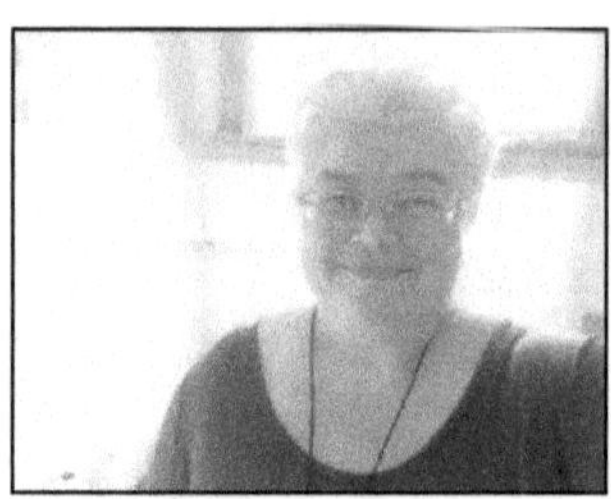

Angela Garry spent 25 years working in administrative roles – 18 of those as a Personal Assistant. After two years of ill health from 2012-2014 and struggling to remain in her really full-on full-time job in a busy school in Nottingham, England, she went through the process of asking herself all of the questions in this book, to decide for herself.

Weighing up the pros and the cons on all sides, Angela decided that it was time to go – and she left her job in February 2014. Much as she loved her job, her physical health simply didn't allow her to continue working the 10 to 12 hour days that the role required and she was unable to perform to the best of her ability.

Since then, Angela has worked part-time from her home office, editing a magazine for PAs working in education, and travelling around the world to deliver training, mentoring and coaching to over 5,100 PAs globally. She is also a prolific author, having written 27 books (so far!) for children and adults, and edited a further 22 for other authors, via her publishing brand Pica Books.

In September 2020 Angela moved home from the UK to Spain where her heath is improving greatly from the change in climate, and where she continues to work part-time from her new home.

Making the difficult decision to leave her job in 2014 was one of the best things she's done.